PHYSICAL FUNCTIONS
OF SKIN

THEORETICAL AND EXPERIMENTAL BIOLOGY

An International Series of Monographs

CONSULTING EDITOR

J. F. Danielli

State University of New York at Buffalo, Buffalo, New York, U.S.A.

PHYSICAL FUNCTIONS
OF SKIN

R. T. TREGEAR

Department of Zoology
University of Oxford, England

1966
ACADEMIC PRESS
LONDON and NEW YORK

ACADEMIC PRESS INC. (LONDON) LTD.
Berkeley Square House
Berkeley Square
London, W.1

U.S. Edition published by
ACADEMIC PRESS INC.
111 Fifth Avenue
New York, New York 10003

Library of Congress Catalog Card Number: 65-18445

PRINTED IN GREAT BRITAIN
BY THE ALDEN PRESS, OXFORD

Preface

The skin is a fascinating study. It can be thought of in several different ways; the biochemist sees it as an assembly of enzymes, the cytologist as an assembly of cell types, the anatomist as a formed structure. The physiologist looks at the functions of the formed structure; this is the theme of the present book.

The main functions of skin are to keep foreign chemicals out, to regulate heat loss, to resist mechanical shocks, and to absorb radiation. In performing these functions the skin acts as a passive, physical structure; all its reactions obey the single classical law of an inert object, "the change produced is proportional to the force producing it". Therefore the physical functions of skin can be empirically described in terms of the various proportionality constants which result from the use of the law: permeability coefficient, thermal conductance, absorbance, elastic modulus, etc.

Once the various functions have been expressed in these proper empirical terms it is possible to travel further, and attempt to explain the empirical terms themselves in terms of the skin's structure. First the function can be assigned to a particular layer of the skin, e.g. permeability is dependent on the keratinized epidermis, elasticity on the dermis. Then the molecular component within that layer may be sought. This is where real difficulties begin to arise, and we reach the limits of our current knowledge. Some functions are mediated by small molecules whose properties are well known, such as the thermal insulation by air or the infrared absorption by water. Others are mediated by the formed protein structures, and relatively little is known of the properties of these macromolecules. Nevertheless, a molecular explanation must be attempted, such as the assignment of permanent stretch to a slip between collagen filaments, or of chemical permeation to the movement of molecules between filaments of α-keratin. Once obtained, the viewpoint of the physiologist links up with those of the cytologist, the anatomist and the biochemist; one knows what the molecules do, while the others know how they are made.

Of the five functions discussed in this book four are restrictive; the skin is adapted to restrict the impact of electricity, radiation, chemicals and force on the body. The last function is regulative; skin can increase or decrease heat flow, at the will of its neural commands. The present description is concerned only with the skin's response, and not the command system.

This book was conceived, and partially written, while I was working at the Chemical Defence Experimental Establishment, Porton, Wilts. Many people there helped me: I wish particularly to thank Mr. Mark Ainsworth for his advice and encouragement, Mr. Peter Dirnhuber for his enthusiastic co-operation, Messrs. A. C. Allenby, J. Edginton and J. A. Fletcher for their assistance, and Dr. W. S. S. Ladell for his support. I should also like to thank

Professor J. W. S. Pringle for allowing me time to finish writing the book after I had moved to Oxford.

I am grateful to Professor G. Causey and Dr. R. D. Harkness for permission to reproduce illustrations from their work.

July 1966   R. T. TREGEAR

Contents

CHAPTER 1

Molecular Movement
The Permeability of Skin

The outside surface of skin is only slightly permeable. Diffusion through it is much slower than through connective tissue or across the surface of capillaries. Skin permeability is now being studied systematically in several laboratories, so that there are many more data than were available to previous reviewers (Calvery *et al.*, 1946; Rothman, 1954; Griesemer, 1959; Malkinson and Rothman, 1962). The first part of the review is divided into three sections, each dealing with one way of looking at the subject. The first section is an empirical statement of the speeds of penetration of different substances, and of the factors which affect these. The second section is a discussion of the relative importance of different histological structures in determining the impermeability of skin. The third section contains a brief description of physical diffusion theories, with evidence as to their relevance to the problem.

It is unfortunate that these three aspects have to be so separated: in an ideal description the physical theory would explain completely the empirical data in terms of the structural element which was known to be the impermeable part. This ideal state has not yet been reached, and the three aspects remain as separate entities.

EMPIRICAL DESCRIPTION

METHODS

Skin permeability has been studied for more than fifty years, and an enormous mass of qualitative data are available, of the kind "A produces a more intense effect, more rapidly than B". Such data are theoretically useless because it is impossible to correlate one set of observations with another; there is no common standard of reference. Recent observers have expressed their results in a quantitative form (e.g. "10 μmoles of A penetrated 25 cm^2 of skin in 8 h from an 0·1 M aqueous solution"). Hence a penetration rate can be deduced for the substance. If, and only if, Fick's law of diffusion holds, these penetration rates can be compared and so the results of different observers can be correlated. Two technical developments in particular have contributed to this improvement: the use of excised skin in diffusion cells, and the use as penetrants of chemicals labelled with radioactive isotopes.

The Use of Excised Skin

Dead skin retains its impermeability. Burch and Winsor (1946) showed this directly for water, and Dirnhuber and Tregear (1960) for tri-n-butyl phosphate; the similarity between the results from intact animals and excised skin (Table III) confirms the point. Excised skin can therefore be used for

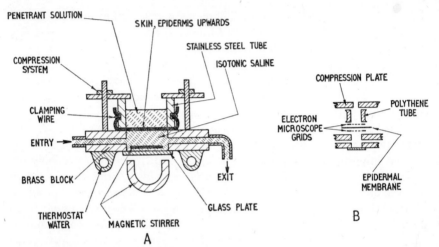

FIG. 1. Diffusion cells, as used for the measurement of penetration by isotope-labelled chemicals through (A) skin or (B) epidermal membranes.

permeability measurements without attempting to keep its cells alive. Some observers have continued observations on excised skin for many days, without noticeable change in the results (e.g. Bettley and Donoghue, 1960). To avoid bacterial contamination it is usual to introduce traces of antibiotics into the system.

The chief advantage of diffusion cells over the use of intact animals or men is in the ease of measurement of the penetrant. The penetrant can be removed from the undersurface of the skin into fluid, usually saline, bathing the surface (Fig. 1) and thus measured without the problems of dilution, distribution and destruction in the body system (Ainsworth, 1960). Alternatively, it may be measured within the dermis, by removal of the tissue after the experiment (e.g. Blank and Gould, 1962). This has the advantage that substances which adhere to the dermis and cannot be washed off in saline can be detected, but the disadvantage that the time-course of penetration cannot be studied.

One practical difficulty in the use of diffusion cells is edge-effect, the movement of penetrant sideways round and through the clamping device. A variety of satisfactory techniques have been used to avoid such leakage. When measuring water loss from the skin surface by weighing the entire cell, a procedure first used by Burch and Winsor (1944) and thereafter by many other observers (cf. Table IIIA), edge-effect is particularly awkward. Isherwood (1963) has devised a novel way of avoiding it.

Penetrant which is collected in saline beneath the dermis has to pass through the full thickness of the dermis, whereas in life it is probably picked up mostly near the dermo-epidermal junction, because the capillary network is most developed there (Krogh, 1922). The dermis is very permeable to aqueous solutes (Treherne, 1956; Burch and de Pasquale, 1962), so that for such substances passage through the dermis is rapid. However, for substances which are only sparingly soluble in water the dermis can present a large diffusional resistance. This has two effects: penetration takes a long time to develop, and the steady penetration rate achieved is lower than that in life (Dirnhuber and Tregear, 1960). This is the principal disadvantage of the diffusion cell. It can be overcome by using epidermis separated from dermis in the cell (Fig. 1B; Bettley and Donoghue, 1960; Marzulli, 1962). Unfortunately such tissue is very fragile, and subject to artifact due to holes appearing at the hair follicles, so that for routine tests of permeability under varying conditions (a major use of the technique; Tregear, 1964b) it is better to use full-thickness skin.

In summary, excised skin diffusion cells are easy to use, and capable of producing rapid, reproducible results. Their validity depends on three assumptions.

1. No living process affects the skin's impermeability.
2. The dermis does not affect penetration.
3. The skin surface conditions are similar to those in life. Because one can rarely, if ever, be certain that these assumptions are completely justified, it is always desirable to check important findings *in vivo*.

The perfused skin preparation described by Kjaersgaard (1954), which consists of a flap of thigh skin supplied by the saphenous artery and vein with remarkably little collateral circulation, may be used for skin permeability measurements (Ainsworth, 1960). It is particularly useful for investigating the effect of circulatory changes on penetration. The preparation is not simple or reproducible enough for use as a routine procedure.

The Use of Radioisotopes

A large variety of chemical and auto-assay methods have been used to detect or measure skin penetration. Some details of the most important methods are shown in Table I. The only quantitative method which compares

TABLE I. *The detection of skin penetrants*

Technique	Range of application
A. *In vivo*	
1. Fluorimetry: body uptake	Used for salicylates (Cotty *et al.*, 1960). Potentially applicable to many dyes. Quantitative: dependent on knowledge of distribution and destruction of compound in the body
2. Radioisotope emission (a) Loss from skin surface	Used for alkyl phosphates (Tregear, 1961), insecticides (Fredriksonn, 1962a), ionic solutions (Wahlberg and Skog, 1962), and corticosteroids (Malkinson, 1958). Quantitative: restricted to high or medium energy β-emitters
(b) Appearance in blood and urine	Used for iodine (Tas and Feige, 1958), borate (Freimuth and Fisher, 1958), tricresyl phosphate (Hodge and Sterner, 1943), water influx (De Long *et al.*, 1954) and many other compounds. Quantitative: knowledge of distribution within body required. No restriction on type of emission (H3 usable)
3. Gravimetry	Used for whole body loss (Zollner *et al.*, 1955) or from restricted area (Heerd and Ohara, 1960; Buettner, 1953). Quantitative: restricted to vaporization of water
4. Anticholinesterase activity	Used for eserine (Valette *et al.*, 1954), sarin (Blank *et al.*, 1958b) and parathion (Vandekar *et al.*, 1963). Quantitative: restricted to anticholinesterase compounds
5. Local anaesthesia	Used for procaine derivatives (Monash, 1957). Qualitative: restricted to anaesthetics
6. Infrared spectrometry	Used for small area loss of water vapour (Albert and Palmes, 1951)
7. Rubefacience and skin blanching	Used for histamine (Shelley and Melton, 1949), corticosteroids (McKenzie and Stoughton, 1962) and nicotinates (Stoughton and Cronin, 1962). Qualitative: restricted to vaso-active substances

Table I—*continued*

B. *In vitro* (all quantitative)

1. Fluorimetry	Used for salicylates (Loveday, 1961)
2. Radioisotope emission	Used for a large variety of substances (Tregear, 1964b; Treherne, 1956). With the advent of tritiated material, suitable for nearly all substances
3. Gas chromatography	Used for aliphatic alcohols (Blank and Scheuplein, 1964). Suitable for substances of boiling point < 350° C
4. Weight loss	Used for water vaporization (Isherwood, 1963; Burch and Winsor, 1944). Restricted to water movement

in sensitivity to radioisotope assay is fluorimetry. This is satisfactory, but is restricted to a limited class of penetrants. The great advantages of the use of radioisotopes are (a) that the penetrant is readily detected and measured in very small amounts, and (b) that, with the introduction of tritium and carbon labels, practically any penetrant may be used.

Radioisotopes can be used in two separate ways: to detect loss from the skin surface, or gain to the body system. For the first, the isotope should emit a medium or high-energy β particle: if the energy is low the particle will be absorbed within the epidermis, so that reduction in count might mean removal by the circulation or merely movement within the epidermis. Some previous measurements suffer from this ambiguity (e. g. Malkinson, 1960). γ-Emission is also undesirable, because removal from the skin to the rest of the body will not necessarily remove the count, as the γ-particle can penetrate a considerable depth of tissue or shielding material. Two further restrictions to its use are that the penetrant can be only slightly volatile, otherwise evaporative loss is large relative to penetration and it must be presented as a thin film on the skin surface, since the penetration is seen as a percentage reduction in the counting and very small percentage reductions cannot be detected. A more detailed description of the details of this technique is given elsewhere (Tregear, 1961).

The conditions for the second method are completely different. As much material may be put on the skin as is desired (consistent with radiological safety) and the type of emission from the isotope is immaterial. However, one requires to measure the whole systemic uptake from the skin source. This can be done using a whole body monitor, if such is available, and the emission is sufficiently penetrating. Otherwise it is necessary to digest the whole animal or take samples from it. The former is tedious, and gives only one value per animal, not a time-series. The latter requires a knowledge of the fate of the chemical ingested. If the urinary excretion of the penetrant is known to be very rapid, urine samples suffice. Alternatively, if its volume of distribution within the body is known, blood samples suffice.

These two developments, the use of radioisotopes and of excised skin, have produced a mass of published quantitative data on skin permeability (Table III), and allow one to obtain data on any desired substance as required. It is from such data that the general pattern of skin penetration, and the factors affecting it, are derived.

THE PATTERN OF SKIN PENETRATION

When an exogenous substance is applied to skin, alone or in solution, it only reaches the circulation or, in the case of a diffusion cell, the washing saline gradually; the rate of transfer through the skin rises to reach a steady rate (Fig. 2). This steady penetration rate is maintained thereafter indefinitely,

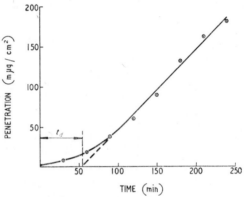

FIG. 2. Penetration of Na$^+$ ions through excised human skin (Thiersch graft) from ^{24}Na labelled 0·9% NaCl on the epidermal surface.

provided (a) that a constant concentration of the penetrant is maintained on the skin, and (b) that the penetrant, or its vehicle, does not attack the skin surface.

The time taken to reach this dynamic equilibrium (or state of constant motion) is given by the delay period, t_d (Fig. 2). The steady state itself is defined by the steady penetration rate r (the slope of the straight line in Fig. 2), whose units are mass per unit time and area (e.g. μmoles/cm^2 h; μg/cm^2 min). The steady penetration rate is the basic parameter required for measurement of skin permeability.

The steady penetration rate has been shown to be proportional to the concentration of penetrant applied to the skin, in a large variety of cases (Table II). Since the circulation beneath the skin, whether natural or artificial, is sufficient to remove the penetrant rapidly from beneath the epidermis (p. 14), this proportionality expresses the simple law of diffusion that the speed of movement is proportional to the driving force, the concentration difference (Fick's law). The proportionality breaks down when a high concentration of penetrant is applied to the skin. Two separate effects may combine to cause this breakdown: interaction between penetrant and skin, e.g. mercuric ion

TABLE II. *Experimental cases where Fick's law holds*

Penetrant	Concn. range	Vehicle	Skin**	Author
Butanol, pentanol	0·1–0·2 M	0·85 % Saline	Human (E)	Blank and Scheuplein (1964)
Pentanol	1–2 M	Olive oil	Human (E)	Blank and Scheuplein (1964)
Salicylic acid	2·5–20 %	Mineral oil	Rabbit (I)	Cotty *et al.* (1960)
Ethanol etc.	0·01–0·05 M	Water	Rabbit (E)	Treherne (1956)
K$^+$ in KCl	0·01–1·0 %	Water	Rabbit (E)	Tregear (1962)
Tri-n-butyl phosphate	0·1–10 %	Propylene glycol, liquid paraffin	Rabbit (E)	Tregear (unpublished)
Hg^{++} in HgCl$_2$	0·1–1 %	Water	Guinea-pig (I)	Wahlberg *et al.* (1961)
Water (evaporation)*			Man (I)	Kerslake *et al.* (1956)
			Man (I)	Heerd and Ohara (1962)
			Man (E)	Berenson and Burch (1951)
			Man (I)	Zollner *et al.* (1955)

* Evaporation rate $\propto$ difference between s.v.p. at skin surface temperature and v.p. of air.

** E, Excised skin; I, intact animal measurement.

(Wahlberg and Skog, 1962), and change of chemical activity in the applied vehicle, e.g. aliphatic alcohols (Blank and Scheuplein, 1964).

When Fick's law holds, the permeability of the skin to the given penetrant molecule may be completely defined by the ratio of the steady penetration rate (r) to the concentration applied (C), the "permeability constant", p:

$$p = \frac{r}{C} \qquad (1)$$

The units of this parameter are length per unit time (e.g. μcm/min; cm/sec $\times 10^{-8}$). Its meaning can be visualized as a depth of applied solution cleared of the penetrant per unit time. Permeability constants may be compared between penetrants, skins and conditions of measurement, and are the only way of relating the observations of different workers. In Table III those

TABLE III. *Permeability constants* (p) *of skin to different molecules, calculated from published data*
E, Excised skin; I, intact animal or man.

Penetrant	Skin species	$p(\mu cm/min)$	Author
A. Water			
Evaporation from excised skin (E)	Man	18	Bettley and Donoghue (1960)
		100–120	Burch and de Pasquale (1962)
		5	Onken and Moyer (1963)
		1–20	Mali (1955)
	Rat	8	Isherwood (1963)
Evaporation from small region of body (I)	Man	25–130	Burch and Winsor (1944)
		5–100	Ikeuchi and Kuno (1927)
		10–20	Pinson (1942)
		25	Craig (1956)
		20	Heerd and Ohara (1962)
		200	McDowell *et al.* (1954)
		30	Buettner (1953)
Evaporation from whole body (I)	Man	15–30	Kerslake *et al.* (1956)
		10	Hancock *et al.* (1929)
		140	Jores (1930)
		15	Jores (1931)
Influx in air	Man (I)	10 ⎫	
	Rat (I)	5 ⎬ De Long *et al.* (1954)	
	Mouse (I)	20 ⎪	
Influx in water	Man (I)	20 ⎭	
	Man (E)	45 ⎫ Tregear (1964b)	
	Rabbit (E)	147 ⎭	
B. Ions in aqueous solution			
Laurate (0·005 M Na laurate)	Man (E)	20 ⎫ Blank and Gould (1959)	
Dodecyl (0·005 M Na dodecyl SO₄)	Man (E)	< 0·5 ⎭	
Borate (10 % boric acid)	Man (I)	< 0·6	Draize and Kelley (1959)
Aluminium (20 % AlCl (OH)₂)	Man (E)	0·02–0·12	Blank *et al.* (1958c)
Mercuric (1–10 mg/ml HgCl₂)	Guinea-pig (I)	15–45	Wahlberg *et al.* (1961)
Chromate (0·02–0·4 M)	Guinea-pig (I)	20–30	Wahlberg and Skog (1963)
Potassium (1·2 % KCl)	Rabbit (I)	52 ⎫	
	Man (I)	1·1 ⎬ Tregear (1966a)	
Bromide (1·6 % NaBr)	Rabbit (E)	53 ⎪	
	Man (E)	0·3 ⎭	
Palmitate (0·04 M)	Man (E)	0·7 ⎫ Bettley (1963)	
Laurate (0·04 M)	Man (E)	50 ⎭	

Table III—*continued*

C. Covalent substances in aqueous solution

Glucose	Rabbit (E)	0·9	⎫
Urea	Rabbit (E)	3	⎪
Methanol	Rabbit (E)	50	⎪
Ethanol	Rabbit (E)	60	⎬ Treherne (1956)
Ethyl iodide	Rabbit (E)	100	⎪
Glycerol	Rabbit (E)	5	⎪
Thiourea	Rabbit (E)	4	⎭
Ethylene bromide	Rabbit (E)	6	⎫
Ethyl phosphate	Rabbit (E)	26	⎬ Tregear (1964b)
Thioglycollic acid	Rabbit (E)	110	⎭
Ethanol	Man (E)	4	⎫
n-butanol	Man (E)	43	⎪
i-butanol	Man (E)	9	⎬ Blank and Scheuplein (1964)
n-pentanol	Man (E)	100	⎭
Salicylic acid	Pig ear (E)	300–600	Loveday (1961)
Human serum albumen	Rabbit (I)	0·015	Tregear (1966b)

D. Organic liquids, undiluted

p-Cymene	Mouse (I)	4·2	Wepierre (1963)
Tri-ethyl phosphate	Rabbit (E)	2·0	Tregear (1964b)
Tri-n-propyl phosphate	Man (E)	0·8	⎫ Marzulli (1962)
Tri-n-butyl phosphate	Man (E)	0·2	⎭
	Rabbit (I)	2·2	⎫ Tregear (1960)
	Pig (I)	0·3	⎭
Paraoxon	Cat (I)	0·2	Fredriksonn (1962a)
Parathion	Cat (I)	1·5	Fredriksonn (1962b)
Sarin	Cat (I)	30	Fredriksonn (1958)
	Rabbit (I)	5	Blank et al. (1958b)
	Man (E)	0·2–2	Blank et al. (1957)
Tricresyl phosphate	Rat (E)	0·004	Tregear (1964b)
Methyl salicylate	Man (I)	3	Wurster and Kramer (1961)
	Rabbit (I)	13	Cotty et al. (1960)

E. Solutes in organic solvents

2 % Parathion in propylene glycol	Rat (I)	2–4	Vandekar et al. (1963)
5 % Paraoxon in xylene	Rat (E)	12	⎫
5 % Tricresyl phosphate in xylene	Rat (E)	0·5	⎪
0·1 % Triethyl phosphate in glycol salicylate	Rabbit (E)	1·5	⎬ Tregear (1964b)
0·1–10 % Tri-n-butyl phosphate in			⎪
(a) glycol salicylate	Rabbit (E)	2·6	⎪
(b) propylene glycol	Rabbit (E)	2·0	⎭
1 % Salicylic acid in polyethylene glycol	Pig ear (E)	6	Loveday (1961)
paraffin	Pig ear (E)	30	
aqueous emulsions	Pig ear (E)	40–100	

measurements which can be turned into permeability constants are assembled. The first section is devoted to the movement of water. Most measurements have concerned the outward loss to air ("insensible water loss") through human skin, but a few have been made of influx from humid air, or from water itself, using deuterium or tritium oxide. In calculating the permeability constant from the data on evaporation, a vapour pressure difference of 40 mm Hg (i.e. difference between dry air and water at the normal skin surface temperature, 32° C) has been considered equivalent to a liquid concentration difference of 1 g/cm^3. The proportionality of vapour loss to vapour pressure difference is well established so that Fick's law may be applied (Table II). The similarity between the permeability constants derived from the evaporative case and the flux under liquid water indicates that the process of diffusion is the same in the two cases, although somewhat higher values under the liquid are to be expected as the skin surface will be more hydrated when covered with water than in air (cf. p. 17). The large reservoir capacity of the skin surface layers for water probably accounts for part of the large variation observed in the work on evaporation.

The second section of Table III is concerned with ions in aqueous solution. The data available are fragmentary, and in some cases require several assumptions before they can be reduced to the form of permeability constants. Thus in Blank's technique the overnight dermal uptake was measured, and one has to assume (a) that the concentration beneath the epidermis remained negligible relative to the applied concentration, and (b) that penetration continued at a steady rate during this period. Draize and Kelley's observations are included as an example of the type of calculation which can be made from some of the older data, but which require so many assumptions that their value is dubious. These authors found that not more than 4 mg borate per kg body weight appeared in rabbits 10% of whose surface had been covered with 10% boric acid solution for 24 h. If the rabbits weighed 2 kg, the area was approx. 100 cm^2, and penetration was less than 8 mg. If penetration was at a steady rate it was less than 0·06 μg/cm^2 min, or for 10% solution, 0·6 μcm/min. The other measurements require no assumptions other than Fick's law.

The table shows that several ions, of either sign, will penetrate skin nearly as rapidly as water, and as rapidly as many covalent substances (Table IIIC). The "impermeability of skin to ions" quoted by earlier authors (cf. Rothman, 1954) therefore does not hold as a general principle. However, some ions obviously do not penetrate skin well (an impression strengthened by many qualitative observations, e.g. Mali et al., 1963). Human skin is much less permeable to ions than rodent skin or pig skin (cf. Fig. 3); this is confirmed by its electrical properties (Chapter 2). Laurate probably attacks the skin surface (p. 21).

Skin penetration by covalent substances in aqueous solution has been studied by relatively few observers. No assumptions other than Fick's law were required in deriving the data of Table IIIC. Apart from the very low value for the macromolecule, albumen, the lowest values are those for glucose and urea (confirmed by Vinson, unpublished observations). The high values for thioglycollic acid and salicylic acid may reflect their interaction with the skin. There is no consistent relationship between oil solubility of the penetrant and its penetration rate (note the low value for ethylene bromide).

The penetration of skin by industrial solvents and insecticides has produced a larger mass of data on the movement of organic liquids through skin (Table IIID). The remarkable thing about these data is that they are nearly all lower than the values for aqueous solutes, although some of the liquids used were miscible with water (e.g. ethyl phosphate). The very low value for tricresyl phosphate is consistent with the earlier observations of Hodge and Sterner (1943), and with observations on intact animals; either skin is remarkably impermeable to this chemical, or it interacts with the skin surface.

Solutes in organic liquids show a similar range of permeability constants to the organic liquids themselves (Table IIIE), with the exception of salicylic acid; it is uncertain whether Loveday's high figures are due to the use of pig ear skin or salicylic acid.

The overall range of permeabilities observed to different substances is very large (0·004–600 μcm/min). However, most of the aqueous solutes lie in the range 3–60 μcm/min, and most of the non-aqueous materials in the range 0·2–10 μcm/min. A substance of small molecular weight whose penetration through skin had not been measured might reasonably be expected to penetrate skin at a speed within these ranges.

The delay before the steady penetration rate is reached (t_d; Fig. 2) may be combined with the steady rate to give an estimate of the capacity of the membrane which restricts penetration (p. 38). The capacity of the membrane (*l*) is related to permeability constant and delay time by the equation

$$l = kpt_d$$

where k is a constant, with values of 4 or 6 in different model systems (Appendix I).

Reliable measurements of t_d are very few, because (a) the measurements on excised skin are useless for this purpose as the dermis prolongs the delay period (Dirnhuber and Tregear, 1960), and (b) the delay period *in vivo* is so short that it is not easily measured. A few values for alkyl phosphates are shown in Table IV; there is an indication that a larger capacity is available to an aqueous solution than to undiluted alkyl phosphate, or to paraoxon.

Passive Nature of the Permeability Barrier

There are three reasons for believing that the movement of molecules across the skin is by passive diffusion. Firstly, the impermeability of skin remains long after the skin has been removed from the animal (e.g. Burch and Winsor, 1946; Ainsworth, 1960); secondly, Fick's law is obeyed, except by substances which are likely, on chemical grounds, to react with the skin surface; and thirdly, there is strong evidence that the diffusional resistance is in the stratum corneum which consists of highly differentiated and metabolically inactive cells (p. 22).

There are two possible exceptions to this: sodium ions and water may be actively pulled into the skin (p. 46).

TABLE IV. *The capacity of the barrier layer to alkyl phosphates and paraoxon*

Substance	t_d (min)	p (μcm/min)	$6pt_d$ (μ)	Author
Tri-n-butyl phosphate				
Rabbit (I)	15	2·2	2·0	Tregear (1960)
Pig (I)	80	0·34	1·6	Tregear (1960)
Pig (perfused)	20	0·15	0·2	Ainsworth (1960)
Tri-n-propyl phosphate				
Man (E, epidermis)	c.10	0·4–4	0·2–2·4	Marzulli (1962)
Tri-ethyl phosphate in aqueous solution				
Man (E, epidermis)	5	30	9	Tregear (unpublished)
Paraoxon (cat, I)	10	0·2	0·1	Fredriksonn (1962a)

FACTORS AFFECTING THE PERMEABILITY OF SKIN

Variations in the Skin

Species

There is a definite and reproducible relationship between the permeabilities of skins of different species. The most complete data available are shown in Fig. 3. Rabbit skin is consistently more permeable than that of other rodents, pigs or men. Human skin is usually the least permeable. It is particularly impermeable to sodium and other common ions.

Age

The only available detailed study of the change in skin permeability as an animal develops was made on rats by Mr. G. Hunt in this laboratory; Fig. 4 illustrates his results, which are unpublished. The impermeability of skin appears during the later stages of foetal development and the first few days after birth; it continues to rise after the epidermis appears histologically mature, i.e. when the stratified squamous layer is fully developed.

Region of the body

The variation of insensible water loss with site on the human body was studied by Ikeuchi and Kuno (1927) and by Burch and Sodemann (1944). Ikeuchi and Kuno found the palm and sole the most permeable, followed by

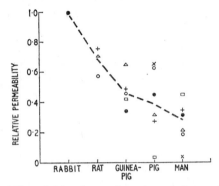

FIG. 3. The permeability of skin of several species, relative to that of the rabbit, for water (●), 5% aqueous thioglycollic acid (○), Na⁺ as 0·9% aqueous NaCl (×), 5% paraoxon in xylene (△), undiluted ethylene bromide (+) and tricresyl phosphate (□). The line is drawn through the mean value for each species. (From Tregear, 1964b.)

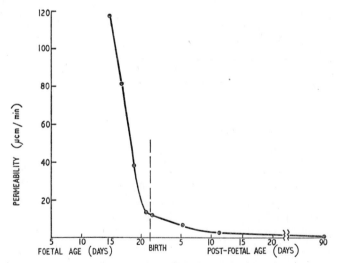

FIG. 4. Permeability of excised rat skin to 5% triethyl phosphate in aqueous solution.

the forehead, cheek and back of the hand, and then the other surfaces. Burch and Sodemann found a similar order: hand > foot > hand > arm > leg > trunk. Mali (1955) also found that palmar skin was more permeable to water *in vitro* than trunk skin.

On the other hand, iodine penetrates palmar skin at only one-third of the rate through forearm skin *in vivo* (Tas and Feige, 1958), and tri-n-butyl phosphate penetrated plantar skin *in vitro* much more slowly than skin from other regions (Marzulli, 1962). Marzulli also showed that postauricular and scrotal skin were the most permeable to tributyl phosphate, and Blank *et al.* (1961) showed that excised scrotal skin was more permeable than abdominal skin to hydrogen sulphide, salicylic acid or water vapour.

Local circulation and retention

The major barrier to diffusion through skin is in the outside layers of the epidermis (p. 21). It follows that changes in the circulation, below the

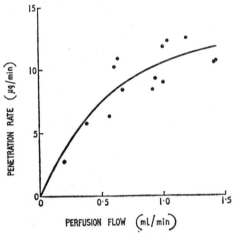

Fig. 5. The penetration of tri-n-butyl phosphate through perfused pig skin, related to the perfusion rate. The results from eight experiments are included.

epidermis, should theoretically have little effect on penetration unless the flow of blood is drastically reduced. This suggestion is supported by results from perfused skin (Kjaersgaard, 1954). The normal blood flow through the saphenous vein of a preparation of pig thigh skin before cutting the artery is in the region of 1 ml/min. Variations in the perfusion rate at and above this level have only a small effect on the penetration of tri-n-butyl phosphate through the skin and into the venous effluent (Fig. 5). Below a flow of 0·5 ml/min, however, the penetration rate drops sharply.

The local action of a skin penetrant should theoretically depend upon the speed at which it is removed by the circulation. The large area of capillary bed available, 1–2 cm²/cm² of skin in man (Krogh, 1922), indicates that removal should be rapid if all the capillaries are open. Intradermally injected aqueous solutes are removed in approx. 10 min (Helde and Seeberg, 1953). Experiments on perfused skin indicate a similar time for the dermal transit of alkyl phosphates arriving percutaneously; rise in perfusion rate causes a transient pulse of penetrant in the effluent for about this period.

Substances which interact with skin components would, of course, be retained in the skin much longer.

Skin surface temperature

The diffusional resistance is in the outer 0·1 mm of the skin, so that in a sparsely haired mammal (man or pig) its temperature varies greatly with environmental conditions. The temperature coefficient of penetration rate has been measured for several substances (Table V); it ranges between 1·4 and 3. Thus, in very cold weather, penetration through a pig or man's exposed skin should fall by up to an order of magnitude.

TABLE V. *The dependence of skin permeability upon temperature*

Penetrant	Q_{10}	Temperature range	Author
Sarin (man, E)	2–3	27–37	Blank *et al.* (1957)
Water evaporation (man, I)	2	25–39	Pinson (1942)
Water evaporation (man, E)	1·4	4–36	Mali (1955)
Triethyl phosphate in water (man, E)	2	20–40	Tregear (unpublished)
Ethanol in water (man, E)	2	20–40	Blank and Scheuplein (1964)

Variations in the Penetrant

Volatility

The characteristics of penetration that have been described above are those of liquids or solutes in liquids. Vapours and permanent gases also penetrate skin; the first thing to determine about their passage is whether it is as vapour or dissolved in some skin component.

Water evaporates from skin into dry air at a similar speed to its movement from liquid water inwards (Table IIIA). Also, its volatility is insufficient to account for a vapour flux of the magnitude seen, unless the skin membrane is extremely permeable to vapour (Table VI). For these reasons water almost certainly crosses the barrier layer in liquid form.

The uptake of alkyl phosphates on excised pig skin from the vapour phase has been measured in this laboratory. An initial uptake is seen, which is higher for the more volatile alkyl phosphate (Fig. 6). This is followed by a slower continued uptake which maintains a steady rate for several hours. The early uptake is readily reversible by exposure to air, and is all removed in the first few applications of adhesive tape to the skin; the later uptake is deeper, and not so readily reversed. The simplest interpretation of these data is that alkyl phosphates, like water, are sorbed on to or dissolved into the surface layers of the skin (the initial uptake), and then penetrate through them in this dissolved state (the continued steady rate).

Permanent gases also penetrate skin. The speed of natural exchange of carbon dioxide and oxygen across skin has been measured many times and

TABLE VI. *The permeability of living human skin to gases*
Permeability constants have been calculated for vapour phase transport (p_1) or aqueous phase transport (p_2).

Gas	Pressure difference (mm Hg)	Mass flow ($\mu g\,cm^{-2}\,min^{-1}$)	Permeability (mcm/min) p_1	p_2	Author
O_2 (influx)	110	0·19	0·9	34	Petrun (1961)
CO_2 (efflux)	50	0·30	2·3	3·4	Fitzgerald (1957)
He (efflux)	610	0·007	0·05	5·8	Klocke *et al.* (1963)
N_2 (efflux)	610	0·02	0·02	1·4	Klocke *et al.* (1963)
A (efflux)	610	0·07	0·05	1·6	Klocke *et al.* (1963)
H_2O (efflux)	40	20	480	0·02	Table IIIA; average value for flux

The solubility of each gas in water at skin temperature was derived from standard tables (Kaye and Laby, 1958).

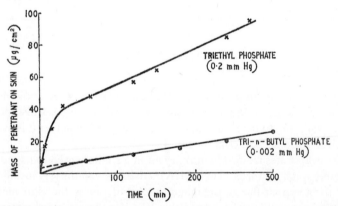

FIG. 6. The uptake of alkyl phosphates on excised pig skin from their vapours; the vapour pressures used are shown.

there are several reviews of the literature (Petrun, 1961; Adams, 1949; Fitzgerald, 1957). Neither of these gas flows obeys Fick's law exactly. Outward loss of oxygen to an atmosphere of nitrogen is negligible, despite its partial pressure in the tissue (Fitzgerald, 1957). This is probably due to the use of oxygen in the epidermis, which lies between the capillaries and the skin surface. Naylor (1959) has noted that the surface oxygen tension under a closed plate changes greatly with blood flow. Carbon dioxide loss is only reversed in sign by an atmospheric pressure greater than 70 mm Hg (Fitzgerald, 1957), presumably also because the epidermal metabolism generates carbon dioxide.

The movement of inert gases across skin is not complicated by these factors: it is therefore much more likely to obey Fick's law. The outward inert gas movements from a lung-generated internal gas pressure have been measured (Klocke *et al.*, 1963). Penetration continues at a steady rate, as in liquid movement. From the steady rates for the various gases permeability constants may be calculated, if one assumes that the gases penetrate either as a gas (p_1 in Table VI) or as a solute in a known solvent (p_2 for water as solvent). Values for carbon dioxide and oxygen are also included in this table, although the Fick's law assumption necessary for the calculation is not justified at low pressures. Water is included to show the very high gas-phase permeability that would be necessary to account for its transfer. For the permanent gases the values of theoretical aqueous-phase permeability constant (p_2) are all much greater than those for known aqueous solutes (Table III). It follows that either the skin is much more permeable to the gas molecules than to other molecules or that the gas molecules pass through in a different solvent or in air. Apart from oxygen all the gases may penetrate in aqueous solutions, for (a) the calculated values of p_2 do not vary widely, (b) all the gas molecules studied are smaller than the other aqueous solutes or water itself, and (c) there are indications that keratinous structures do behave as if they contained very small pores (p. 41). This is at present a very loose argument which requires more experimental data for its determination. Oxygen is very poorly soluble in water, so that its penetration through skin is likely to be in some other skin component or as a gas.

Solvent

It has frequently been shown that the penetration rate of a solute through skin varies with its solvent. The amount of variation is less reliable. Valette *et al.* (1954) and Meyer and Kerk (1959) showed that eserine penetrated rodent skin from aliphatic alcohol or ester solution at a rate dependent on the aliphatic chain length, but the variations in rate indicated were only 2–3 × (these observers worked to an end-point of muscular activity induced by the anticholinesterase, so the results are not immediately related to penetration rate). Tregear (1964b) also found that tri-n-butyl phosphate penetrates skin at very similar rates from different solvents. On the other hand, several observers have found large differences between the penetration from different solvents (Table VII). From these results water often, but not always, appears to enhance skin penetration. This impression is reinforced by the lower permeability of skin to organic liquids than to aqueous solutes (Table IIIC, D). In artificial horn membranes permeability to water vapour has also been shown to vary greatly with the hydration of the tissue (King, 1945). Also from the data in Table VII it appears that tricresyl phosphate actively retards skin penetration.

An exogenous solvent is not essential for penetration to occur. Solids dried on to the skin from a volatile solvent penetrate long after the exogenous solvent has evaporated (Stoughton and Fritsch, 1963; Tregear, 1964b).

TABLE VII. *Variation of permeability of excised skin with solvent applied*

Substance	Solvent	p (μcm/ min)	Author
Triethyl phosphate	Glycol salicylate	1·5	Tregear (1964b)
	Triethyl phosphate	1·9	
	1 : 1 Ethanol-water	15·5	
	Water	25·8	
Tri-n-butyl phosphate	Glycol salicylate	2·6	Tregear (1964b)
	Paraffin	4·6	
	Propylene glycol	2·0	
	Tri-n-butyl phosphate	2·1	
Tri-o-cresyl phosphate	Xylene	0·46	Tregear (1964b)
	Tricresyl phosphate	0·0042	
Paraoxon	Xylene	12·3	Tregear (1964b)
	Tricresyl phosphate	0·7	
Ethylene bromide	Ethylene bromide	4·4	Tregear (1964b)
	Water	5·8	
Ethanol	Water	4	Blank and Scheuplein (1964)
	Olive oil	40	
n-Pentanol	Water	100	Blank and Scheuplein (1964)
	Olive oil	18	
Salicylic acid	Polyethylene glycol	6	Loveday (1961)
	Water	600	

Mass of penetrant available

A steady concentration on the skin surface is necessary for a steady penetration rate. In practical testing of skin penetration the amount of penetrant placed on the skin is often very small, e.g. insecticides (Fredriksonn, 1962a) or steroids (Stoughton and Cronin, 1962). In order to fill the holes in the surface of skin approx. 1 mg/cm^2 liquid must be applied (E. A. Taylor, 1961). Above this amount an applied liquid forms a definite liquid pool on the skin surface, penetration rate is independent of the mass applied (Blank *et al.*, 1957), and the use of the permeability constant is appropriate. Below 1 mg/cm^2 there is no liquid overtly on the surface, and the penetration rate is dependent, linearly, on the mass of penetrant applied (Fig. 7), i.e. the effective concentration available is proportional to the mass. The appropriate parameter is therefore not the permeability constant but the fraction of dose applied which penetrates per unit time (% per min). This point is of great practical importance (Tregear, 1964a).

Molecular weight of penetrant

There appears to be a coarse relationship between molecular size and penetration rate: helium, the smallest molecule tested, passes through the skin the most rapidly of all molecules (Table VI), while human serum albumin passes through the skin very slowly indeed (Table IIIC). Within a smaller range of molecular size, however, there is no correlation between size and rate; other factors are more important.

Even particles of more than macromolecular dimensions will pass through

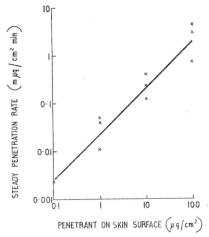

FIG. 7. The relation between penetration of tri-n-butyl phosphate through excised pig skin and the mass of alkyl phosphate applied.

skin slowly: Iunin (1958) reported transference of colloidal or powdered sulphur across rabbit skin, the effectiveness of inunction of metallic mercury is well known (Rothman, 1954), and two observers have found bacteria below the skin after dipping rodents' tails in concentrated bacterial culture (Lizgunova, 1959; Keller, 1958). The actual penetration rates are not calculable at present.

Solubility

The solubility characteristics necessary for a substance to penetrate skin rapidly are still uncertain. Treherne (1956) found a direct relation between the ether : water partition coefficient of an aqueous solute and its permeability constant through rabbit skin. He suggested that a partition coefficient of unity might be the optimum for penetration. There are several other facts which support this hypothesis: triethyl phosphate, which is readily soluble in both oil and water does penetrate skin readily, while Stoughton and his co-workers have shown that the solely water-soluble nicotinic acid and acetyl-salicylic acid penetrate skin very slowly (Stoughton and Fritsch, 1963; Stoughton and Cronin, 1963; Stoughton et al., 1960).

However, at least some ions in aqueous solution penetrate skin as rapidly as other aqueous solutes (Table III) and there are many other semi-quantitative observations of skin penetration by ions (e.g. Norgaard, 1957; Stuttgen and Betzler, 1956; Lotmar, 1958; Tas and Feige, 1958; Mali et al., 1963); ions are barely soluble at all in ether. Also some organic liquids and solutes therein of negligible solubility in water penetrate skin more rapidly than would be expected if they had to diffuse through an aqueous membrane.

Surface Treatments which Affect Skin Permeability

Keratolytics

Alkaline sodium sulphide or thioglycollic acid will attack keratinized epidermal cells, dissolving the keratin (p. 31). They also greatly increase the permeability of epidermal membranes to water or triethyl phosphate (Tregear, unpublished observations), although they do not affect the permeability of skin to water (Berenson and Burch, 1951). The high permeability of skin to thioglycollic acid (Table IIIB) is also probably due to its keratolytic action. There are many different keratolytics whose actions on keratin are described in detail by Mercer (1962).

Organic liquids

Many workers have washed skin with organic solvents before measuring its permeability. They have found very variable effects. Washing the skin surface with ether or petroleum ether had little effect on the permeability of skin to salicylates (Wurster and Kramer, 1961), water (Burch and de Pasquale, 1962) or surfactants (Blank and Gould, 1962; Blank et al., 1964) and epidermal membranes prepared by soaking in petroleum ether for several hours have been found to be as impermeable as whole skin to alkyl phosphate (Marzulli and Tregear, 1961; Marzulli, 1962).

On the other hand, prolonged treatment of skin with acetone, alcohol or hexane (all polar solvents) does greatly increase the permeability of skin to water (Berenson and Burch, 1951; Onken and Moyer, 1963).

Surfactants

Detergent and soap solutions remove some of the amino acid content of the skin surface cells (Blank and Shappiro, 1955). This removal does not appear to have a large effect on skin permeability: Wahlberg et al. (1961)

found only a slight increase of mercuric chloride transfer through skin after washing with soap. On the other hand, surface-active agent actually in the penetrating solution increases skin permeability to water (by a factor of × 3–10; Bettley and Donoghue, 1960; Isherwood, 1963), to glucose (Bettley, 1961) and, from observation of the dermatitis provoked, to nickel ions (Vinson and Choman, 1960). The effects of surfactants on salicylate transfer are disputed: Bettley (1961) noted an increased, Loveday (1961) a decreased permeability on addition of surfactant to the solution. Detergents themselves penetrate skin at rates similar to those of other aqueous solutes (Table IIIB); the most penetrating anion, laurate, also has the largest effect on the permeability to other solutes (Bettley, 1963).

CONCLUSIONS

The skin is appreciably permeable to all the molecules that have been tested. This is a genuine permeability, i.e. a movement through a passive diffusional resistance. The resistance varies widely, depending on the size of the molecule transferred, the nature of the vehicle employed and the state of the skin surface, but it is never negligible and never infinite. The skin behaves as an unspecific barrier, stopping nothing perfectly but slowing transfer of all substances considerably, and is very insensitive to a large variety of chemical insults.

THE STRUCTURAL BASIS OF THE SKIN'S IMPERMEABILITY

If the epidermis is removed from skin, the residual tissue is very permeable to water (Berenson and Burch, 1951), aqueous solutes (Treherne, 1956) and organic liquids (Marzulli, 1962). Isolated human epidermis, which can be separated from the dermis by a variety of chemicals which affect the collagen (Felsher, 1947) by mild heat or ammonia (Baumberger et al., 1941) or by cantharidin (Einbinder and Walzer, 1963), is as impermeable as whole skin to water (Berenson and Burch, 1951; Bettley and Donoghue, 1960) or organic liquids (Marzulli and Tregear, 1961; Marzulli, 1962). The resistance to diffusion through skin, or diffusional barrier, is therefore in the epidermis.

If the surface layers only of the human epidermis are pulled off on adhesive tape (Pinkus, 1952), the permeability of the skin rises greatly, to water (Blank, 1953; Monash and Blank, 1958), procaine derivatives (Monash, 1957), corticosteroids (Malkinson, 1958) and ions (by inference from impedance; Lawler et al., 1960). Biopsy has shown that this process removes only the mature stratified layers of the epidermis (Lobitz and Holyoke, 1954; Lawler *et al.*, 1960); this is because the latex surface of the adhesive tape will only stick to a dry surface, and only the stratified layers are dry (Tregear and Dirnhuber, 1962). As this "stripping" technique causes erythema and a definite epidermal recovery cycle (Hunter and Williams, 1957), it clearly causes changes deeper than the material it removes and is thus not conclusive proof that the barrier lies within the surface layers. However, Blank *et al.* (1958a) showed that cuts which only penetrated the stratum corneum (and caused none of the secondary changes described above) also greatly increased the permeability, as judged by local penetration of sarin. Monash and Blank (1958) and Matoltsy *et al.* (1962) have shown that the impermeability of stripped skin to water returns as the stratum corneum regenerates.

Separated epidermis can be reduced by maceration to a membrane containing only the mature stratified cells; such a membrane retains its low permeability to water (Mali, 1955). The epidermal membranes employed in diffusion cells (e.g. Bettley and Donoghue, 1960) are also free of living cells, for they are retained for several days under unphysiological conditions. A membrane of stratified cells (the "stratum corneum conjunctum" of Szakall) can also be produced by pulling them off the skin surface on adhesive tape. Under favourable conditions (good adhesion and damp skin lower down) this removes whole sheets of cells. If the adhesive used is of the rubber latex type (e.g. Sellotape) the cell sheet has to be separated from it by petroleum ether, or some other organic solvent; if of collagen glue (e.g. Aero Universal glue spread on Whatman No. 41 filter paper) the membranes can be removed in water or saline solution.

All these membranes are very impermeable. Stripped cell sheets are as impermeable as whole skin to alkyl phosphates (Marzulli, 1962).

It is therefore practically certain that the diffusional resistance of the epidermis lies within the stratum corneum, the fully formed keratinized layer of the epidermis.

PARALLEL PATHS

The hair follicles and sweat glands of skin clearly represent potential parallel paths, or short circuits, of the epidermal system. Despite classical dermatological teaching there are several reasons for believing that they are not important routes. Firstly, in man the palmar skin is less permeable to substances (except water) than the rest of the body (p. 13). Yet there are three times as many sweat glands per unit area of palm or sole skin as elsewhere (Szabo, 1962; Kuno, 1956). Secondly, anhydrotic subjects have as large an insensible water loss as normal people (Richardson, 1926). It is therefore unlikely that in the main body surface (excluding the palmar and plantar surfaces) much of the penetrant passes through the sweat glands. In mammals other than the primates, sweat glands open into or just adjacent to the hair follicles, except on the pads and snout, and therefore as a parallel path for penetration can be considered as part of the hair follicles.

In man there are 40–70 hairs/cm^2 on the skin of the trunk and limbs (Szabo, 1962). In most mammals, there are many more: the densely haired rodents have up to 4 000 hairs/cm^2 (Table VIII). In man the invaginated area of stratified epithelium within the hair follicles is small relative to that on the skin surface (Table VIII). A similar calculation for rabbit or horse skin indicates that much more epithelium lines the hair follicles than the surface

TABLE VIII. *Calculated area of invaginated epithelium within hair follicles*

Species	Number (/cm² skin)	Length (cm)	Width (μ)	Relative area*
Man, forearm	60	0·1	50	0·1
Pig, flank	40	0·3	120	0·4
Horse, belly	800	0·3	100	7·5
Rabbit, flank	$\left\{\begin{array}{r} 700 \\ 3000 \end{array}\right.$	0·15 0·15	50 20	$\left.\begin{array}{l} 1\cdot6 \\ 2\cdot8 \end{array}\right\}$ 4·4

* Total area of cylinders of these dimensions per unit area of skin.

The data in this table are derived from measurements from two to four animals and the values are therefore only approximate. They are *not* intended as authoritative biometric data.

of the skin. Thus the potential penetration through hair follicles in densely furred animals, if the penetrant gets down the follicle, is very large even if the rate per unit area of epithelium is no greater than on the surface.

In fact, the permeability of rodent skin to many diverse substances (excluding ions) is 3–5 times that of human skin. This indicates *either* that the rate of penetration of the hair follicle walls is no greater than that of the surface *or* that penetrants do not get down the hair follicles. The penetration of materials down hair follicles has been noted histochemically (Mackee *et al.*, 1945) and autoradiographically (Axelrod and Hamilton, 1947; Wepierre and Valette, 1962; Choman, 1960), so that the second alternative is unlikely to be generally true, although Blank *et al.* (1958a) found little entry of sarin into human hair follicles.

If penetration per unit area of epithelium is similar within and outside the hair follicle, skin penetration in man or pig should be largely via the exposed epidermis, since only a small fraction of the available epithelium is in the hair follicles (Table VIII). This hypothesis has been checked on the pig using tri-n-butyl phosphate. When this material was placed on pig skin it penetrated equally readily whether the area included hair follicles or not (Tregear, 1961).

It is therefore probable that much of the observed penetration, in man or animals, is actual penetration through the stratified system, and not through pilosebaceous "holes" in the system.

SEBUM AS A BARRIER

Most skin, except that of the palms, soles and snout, possesses sebaceous glands; the comparative aspects of sebaceous gland secretion have been studied in detail by Montagna (1963). The glands which are peculiar to mammals reach their greatest development in lemurs and bats, but are present in all mammalian orders. Their morphology is very variable but most glands of the general body surface are simple structures opening into the hair follicles.

The sebaceous secretion reaches the skin surface as a layer of fatty material which, in man, has been estimated as $0.4-4$ μ thick (Table IX). The recovery

TABLE IX. *Mass of sebum on the skin surface of man, and its rate of secretion*

Author	Site	Mass (μg/cm^2)	Rate (μg/cm^{2}min)
Hermann and Prose (1951)	Forehead	200	1·3
	Abdomen	60	—
	Chest	130	—
	Forearm	50	0·3
Kligman (1963)	Abdomen	50	—
Kirk (1948)	Forehead	200–400	—
Strauss and Pochi (1961)	Forehead		
	(adult ♂)	—	1·6
	(juvenile ♂)	—	0·5
Jones *et al.* (1951)	Forearm	45	0·1–1*

* Dependent on mass already on the skin.

from the skin is highly dependent on the method used: solvents may remove sub-surface lipids, while wiping with absorbent paper may not remove all the surface material. Nevertheless, the range of values obtained by different investigators is reasonably consistent. Replacement takes place in 1–6 h; it appears to be a passive matter of continuous secretion and casual removal with no elaborate feedback mechanisms (Kligman, 1963).

The mass of sebum on the skin surface has not been measured in other species. Apart from special cases like the marmoset's belly (Montagna, 1963), visual observation of the skin surface of hairy animals indicates less fat than on human skin: the surface does not reflect light, and appears free of grease.

The surface fat of human skin consists of one-third free fatty acids of high chain length (Nicolaides, 1961), one-third esterified fatty acids, and one-third unsaponifiable material (Mackenna *et al.*, 1950). The free fatty acids are probably formed from the sebum in the ducts of the sebaceous glands (Nicolaides and Wells, 1957). The acidity of the skin surface sebum has been measured many times (Blank, 1939; Draize, 1942; Schirren, 1955; Jolly *et al.*, 1961).

Most recent estimates place the pH in the region 5·0–6·7. Sebum will flow readily on water, but not on dry skin (Jones *et al.*, 1951); it has a high temperature coefficient of viscosity, which amounts to a gradual solidification in the temperature range 15–33° C (Butcher and Cronin, 1949), but in the presence of water remains "liquid" to lower temperatures due to the ready formation of emulsions (Rothman, 1954). It has been suggested by Hermann *et al.* (1952) that these emulsions "change phase" on the skin surface so as to conserve water, but Kligman (1963) has pointed out that they are unstable on the skin surface and have a very transitory existence.

The effect of this thin layer of emulsifiable fat on penetration through skin is probably very slight. Kligman (1963) deliberately added sebum to the surface of epidermal membranes and only found a reduction in water evaporation when 3·5 mg/cm² was added (30 μ thickness)—ten times the maximum observed natural thickness in man. Mild swabbing with acetone or ether has no effect on the water loss through live human skin (Burch and de Pasquale, 1962), and ether swabbing decreased the penetration of salicylic acid (Wurster and Kramer, 1961). Such treatments have been used for quantitative recovery of sebum, so that it is highly probable that the sebum has little effect on skin penetration. More prolonged action of a solvent certainly does increase skin permeability (Onken and Moyer, 1963), but is likely to affect other structures as well as the sebum (Swanbeck, 1959). Theoretically, sebum should only restrict the passage of polar molecules, since such a thin layer forms a negligible diffusional resistance (Higuchi, 1960), and the relatively rapid passage of such polar substances through normal skin (Table III) shows that the sebum does not form a functionally complete lipoidal film over the skin.

After this argument the only remaining source of the diffusional resistance is the stratum corneum, the layer of mature keratinized cells which forms the outer part of the epidermis (Fig. 8).

THE STRATIFIED SQUAMOUS CELL AS A BARRIER

Formation of the Stratum corneum

The epidermis can be considered as a system for the manufacture of horny plates. The life cycle of the human epidermal cell has been worked out by Pinkus (1954). In man most, but not all, of the cell divisions take place in the basal layer of the epidermis; there are some divisions in the spinous layer. In hairy mammals the epidermis is much thinner (Fig. 8) so that it is likely that all the cell divisions are in the basal layer. All epidermal cells, except the melanocytes, are connected by "desmosomes" (Birbeck *et al.*, 1961), structures which have a characteristic banded appearance under the electron microscope (Fig. 9; Odland, 1958) and form the "spines" seen under the light microscope. The desmosomes probably hold the cells together, for Charles and Smiddy

B

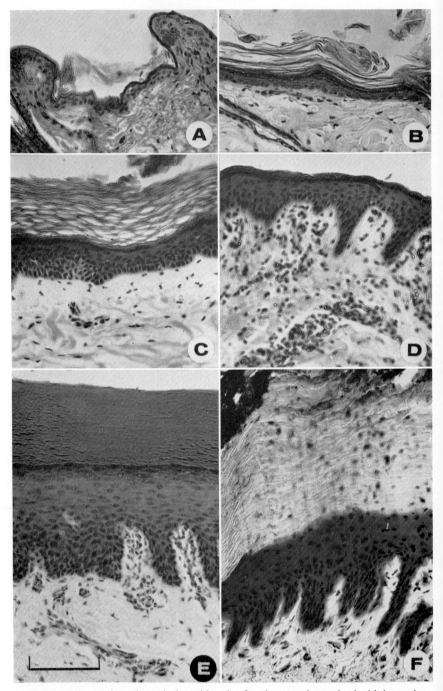

FIG. 8. Cross-sections through the epidermis of various species, stained with haemalum and eosin. A, Cat (back); B, rat (back); C, man (ankle); D, pig (flank); E, guinea-pig (hind pad); F, elephant (knee). Scale 100 μ.

(1957) showed that when the epidermis is fixed under tension they can be seen to connect the internal fibres (tonofilaments) of protein within the cells. As the cells move towards the skin surface they become flattened (Fig. 8) and then fill up with protein granules (keratohyalin). These granules are irregularly

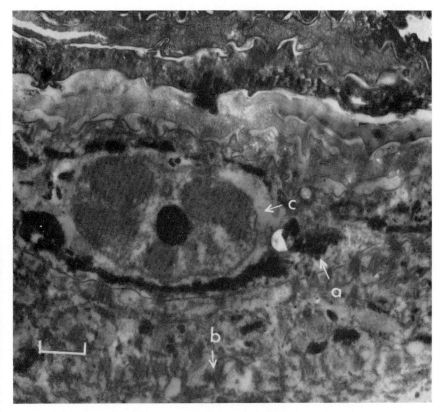

FIG. 9. Electron micrograph of cross-section through the keratinizing cells of the human epidermis. a, Keratohyalin granule; b, desmosome between spinosum cells; c, nucleus of granulosum cell. Scale 1 μ.

associated with the tonofilaments (Mercer, 1962; Brody, 1962). The mitochondria and nuclei of the granulosum cells appear degenerate (Selby, 1957). For a detailed description of the histochemistry of epidermal cells, see Montagna (1962).

Immediately above the granulosum cells lies the stratum corneum, whose cells contain only nuclear and mitochondrial remnants (Horstmann and Dabelow, 1957; Odland, 1960) amongst a mass of keratin. A few transitional cell types have been identified under the electron microscope by Brody (1960) and Zelickson (1961), but the overriding impression is of a rapid change, practically a switch, from the maturing to the mature cell. This is demonstrated dramatically in another keratinous tissue, Henle's layer of the hair, where granular cytoplasm and mature keratin can be seen at opposite ends of the same cell (Mercer, 1962). The immediate source of the fibrous protein, from keratohyalin or tonofilament, remains in dispute (Laden *et al.*, 1957; Charles, 1959; Mercer, 1962).

Each cell is reckoned to take up to 200 days to mature in human epidermis (Pinkus, 1954) but much less in rodents. The life-time of the mature cell is 7–20 days. The process of keratinization is dependent on the presence of the dermis (Dodson, 1963) and is regulated by the local level of vitamin A (Rubin, 1960; Flesch, 1963). When the epidermis is damaged, it regenerates by an organized sequence of mitotic waves (Pinkus, 1952; Cruikshank and Hell, 1963).

Skin keratinization is essentially the same throughout the vertebrates, although the end product differs enormously in appearance and quantity, e.g. teleosts have few mature keratinous cells in their skin (Burgess, 1956), lizards possess an organized cycle of development and desquamation (Poly-akova, 1962), and pachyderms develop extremely thick keratinized layers. A general description of vertebrate skin is given by Biedermann (1928).

Structure of the Mature Cells

The fully keratinized cell of the stratum corneum is a thin, flat, approximately hexagonal plate (Figs. 10–12). In man each plate measures approx. $25 \times 0.5 \, \mu$, except the palmar squames which are much thicker. The plates lie tangential to the skin surface, and their lateral edges interdigitate with adjacent cells (Fig. 12) so as to form laminae, which can lift off intact during histological preparation or on adhesive tape. Several such laminae make up the whole thickness of the stratum corneum; the total number varies widely between regions of the body and between species. The optical microscope reveals little of the internal structure of these cornified plates (Fig. 10; Horst-mann and Dabelow, 1957); the description which follows is based entirely on electron micrographs. Each cell consists of three components: the keratin itself, a non-keratinous shell surrounding it, and the "desmosome" attach-ments to other cells. The keratin is composed of a tightly packed mass of fibrils at 80–100 Å spacing (Brody, 1959; Zelickson, 1961; Horstmann and Knoop, 1958). The centre of each fibril is less osmiophil than the matrix which surrounds it. The fibrils form parallel arrays over distances of up to 7 000 Å (Brody, 1959; Fig. 13) but not across the entire thickness of the cell. Fibrils of similar diameter are found in wool and hair cortical cells (Mercer, 1962). They show a characteristic electron microscope structure (Rogers and Filshie, 1963), and low angle diffraction pattern; from these data several

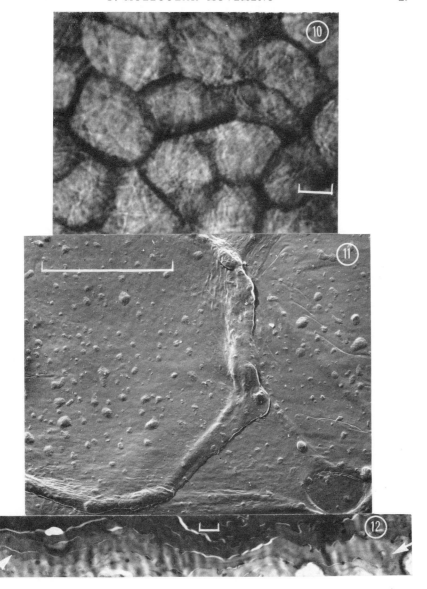

FIG. 10. Optical micrograph of the keratinized cells in a cellular sheet torn off the forearm with adhesive tape and stained with iron haematoxylin. Scale 10 μ.

FIG. 11. Electron micrograph of carbon replica of the surface of a similar cellular sheet. Scale 10 μ.

FIG. 12. Electron micrograph of a cross-section through a keratinized cell, the edges of which are marked by arrows. Scale 1 μ.

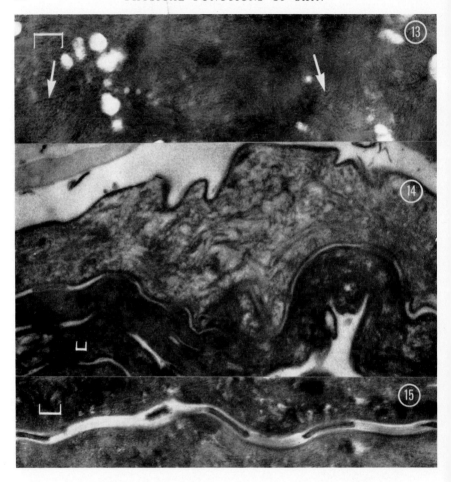

FIG. 13. Fine filamentous structure of keratin in a human palmar keratinized cell. The arrows mark regions in which the filaments were cut in cross-section. Scale 0·1 μ.

FIG. 14. Keratinized cell in which the keratin has broken up, revealing the non-keratinous shell around the cell. Scale 0·1 μ.

FIG. 15. Intercellular bodies (desmosomes) between keratinized cells of human instep skin. A continuous banded structure fills the space between the cells. Scale 0·1 μ.

alternative protein chain packings have been proposed (Lundgren and Ward, 1963).

Around the cell there is a dense osmiophil shell, 100–200 Å thick. It shows no internal structure and remains intact when the keratin breaks up (Fig. 14). The keratin reaches right up to the shell. Outside the shell there is occasionally a thin osmiophil line, particularly when the cell is adjacent to a desmosome;

this may be a plasma membrane (Brody, 1959; Zelickson and Hartmann, 1961). A shell is also found around wool and hair cells (Alexander and Earland, 1950).

Desmosomes are intercellular banded structures seen in many tissues. In the stratum corneum they appear to be extracellular, and consist usually of two 100 Å thick osmiophil bars separated by 200 Å and backed by a "plasma membrane" at double the distance. The whole structure is 350–450 Å across. Desmosomes occur either as isolated structures, with a much thinner intercellular space in the interval between them (Brody, 1959), or as condensations on a continuous, less osmiophil structure (Fig. 15); a similar formation can be seen in the inner root sheath of the hair (Mercer, 1962). The intercellular space in the absence of desmosomes is amorphous and of indefinite thickness; Brody quoted a thickness of 160 Å, but in our observations the space frequently appeared to vanish altogether, presumably due to cell overlap in the section.

The electron microscope picture of the keratinized cell can be related to its chemical properties. The chemistry of wool keratin has received great attention (Mercer, 1962) and as the electron microscope picture of cortical wool cells resembles that of the keratin in epidermal keratinized cells, it is probable that the two structures are similar. Wool keratin can be separated into two components by differential alkaline reduction or acid oxidation: the first, α-keratin, reforms fibres when precipitated and is believed to form the natural keratin fibrils (Lundgren and Ward, 1963). It has a low sulphur content which would explain its low uptake of osmium. The other component, γ-keratin, is a globular protein of high sulphur content which is believed to form the matrix surrounding the α-keratin filaments. There is approximately three times as much α-keratin as there is γ-keratin (Mercer, 1962). Soaking wool in an alchohol–ether mixture changes its X-ray diffraction pattern (Swanbeck, 1959) so that there may also be some lipid within the structure.

If the analogy is correct, these characteristics probably also apply to epidermal keratin. Some component of epidermal keratin is certainly very easily eluted by hydrolysis, for water alone will remove a significant proportion of the amino acids from keratinized epidermal cells (Stüpel and Szakall, 1957).

Both wool and epidermal keratin are highly resistant to the action of proteinases, apart from the specialized keratinases of the clothes-moth larva (Linderstrom-Lang and Duspiva, 1935) and certain fungi (Stahl et al., 1950). The shells of the keratinized cells are far more easily attacked by enzymes: in the hair pancreatin destroys the shells completely leaving sheaves of keratin (Elod and Zahn, 1946). On the other hand, bacterial keratinase does not separate the cells of the stratum corneum (Dobson and Bosley, 1963). Hydrolytic reducing agents do not affect the shell, and "pure" shell preparations can be prepared from skin by such reagents (Matoltsy, 1958; Lagermalm et al.,

1951). These "ghosts" retain the shape of the original cells, and so presumably are fairly rigid. They are composed of protein, of a slightly different amino acid composition than keratin (Matoltsy, 1958). Since the thickness of the ghost shell is 100 Å (Lagermalm et al., 1951), it is probably the same as the osmiophil shell seen under the electron microscope. Because of its chemical properties and its apparent rigidity, it has been suggested that the shell protein chains are cross-linked by quinones, i.e. tanned, but the scarcity of aromatic amino acids in the shell protein analysis (Matoltsy, 1958) makes this unlikely.

The other parts of the system are less easily identified or separated chemically. The electron micrographs give no certainty that a plasma membrane regularly invests the cell, but always show intercellular attachment bodies (desmosomes) and often show a continuous regular set of bands between the cells. It is therefore logical to look for proteophospholipids in extracts of the cells, which might form sets of orientated molecules and give rise to the appearance seen with the electron microscope.

There is little phospholipid in the stratum corneum (0·14% in palm or sole; Kooynan, 1932). This does not mean that there is no phospholipid between the cells, however; there are no viable mitochondria and few cell inclusions in the cornified cell (Selby, 1957; Odland, 1958), and as these are associated with a large proportion of the phospholipid of living cells the low percentage may simply be due to their absence. However, since the volume of intercellular space is approx. 1% of the whole (400 Å channels separating 40 000 Å thick sheets in the palm), the phospholipid could not occupy the whole of it. Periodic acid–Schiff's reagent (PAS) stains the intercellular region, even after the action of diastase. This very unspecific reaction indicates the presence of some acid attached to a polymer (Pearse, 1960) and is often associated with an acid polysaccharide such as hyaluronic acid. Flesch and Esoda (1960, 1962) extracted a hexosamine-containing glycoproteolipid from callus and from psoriatic scales. This could have caused the PAS stain; Brody (1960) has noted that the intercellular space is widened and filled with an electron-dense material in psoriasis. A similar lipoprotein was extracted from hair with polar solvents by Holmes (1961).

Although the quantity of phospholipid or of hexosamine (Smith et al., 1962) present in stratified epidermis is very small, the total quantity of lipid which can be extracted from stratum corneum with ether, 2–4% (Flesch, 1958; Spier and Pascher, 1956), is sufficient to fill the intercellular space. Most of this fat is glyceride, sterol, wax and hydrocarbon (Wheatley and Reinartson, 1959); it contains some very long chain fatty acids (Wheatley et al., 1963). Only 1% is phospholipid.

The desmosomes are unlikely to be a diffusional barrier since there are always ways around them. Their prime function is believed to be adhesion between cells; there are large numbers in the strong callus material of the palm.

Permeability of Laminae within the Stratum corneum

There are structural gradations within the stratum corneum from its granular layer surface to its free surface. Brody (1959) has differentiated at least three types of cells, correlated with depth: he found the finest keratin matrix to exist in the lowest cells. Wolf (1937, 1954) noted four stages in the development of Gram-staining of the squames; the Gram-staining material may be a mucophysaccharide (Flesch and Roe, 1960). The upper layers of keratinous cells are more easily removed on adhesive tape than the lower layers (Fig. 16; for details see Tregear and Dirnhuber, 1962) which adhere

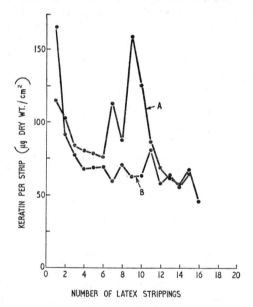

FIG. 16. Mass of keratin removed by successive strippings of the same area of the flexor surface of the forearm in two individuals. A, Conjunctum on tapes 7–11; B, no conjunctum removed. (Tregear and Dirnhuber, 1962.)

together more and hence can be removed as membranes (Szakall, 1955). These gradations indicate that the keratinous cells are changing in their internal structure and in their adhesion as they move outwards. Is there a corresponding change in their diffusional resistance?

When skin is "stripped" with adhesive tape each application of the tape brings off only a small fraction of the total keratin. The particles removed are clumps of cells, usually more than one cell thick but not the full thickness of the stratum corneum (Tregear and Dirnhuber, 1962; Blank et al., 1961). The effect is of a fairly uniform thinning of the stratum by each stripping. It is therefore possible to use this technique as a means of estimating the relative permeability of the different layers removed.

C

Each stripping increases the permeability of the remaining skin to water (Blank, 1953), local anaesthetics (Monash, 1957) and endogenous ions (Lawler *et al.*, 1960). It follows that each stripping *either* removes some of the impermeable material *or* disturbs it lower down. The effect of successive strippings on the permeability increases greatly as the last few layers of stratified cells are removed (see references cited above and Monash and Blank, 1958). This does not necessarily show that the lowest layers are the least permeable; a hyperbolic relation between permeability and thickness remaining would be expected for a uniformly impermeable substance. However, it does show that the lowest layers of the stratum corneum have a large diffusion resistance.

The squamous cell membranes which can be pulled off on adhesive tape usually consist of only the lower layers of the stratum corneum; Szakall (1955) termed the membrane the "stratum corneum conjunctum" as distinct from the "disjunctum" which came off as particles. This distinction is not an absolute anatomical one, for when the surface of the stratum corneum is very dry and its substance wet (as in skin air-dried after some hours under an occlusive dressing), the whole thickness may be removed as a "conjunctum" membrane. The membranes removed sometimes have an impermeability as great, or nearly as great, as that of whole skin (Marzulli, 1962). This indicates that the lower part of the stratum corneum is more impermeable than the upper part.

Another experiment which bears on this point is the mass of penetrant removed with each stripping. If a penetrant is left on the skin for some time, the surface is blotted free of surplus liquid and the skin stripped; most of the penetrant is found near the surface of the stratum corneum (Born, 1958; Goldhamer and Carson, 1963; Fig. 17). This is most easily interpreted as meaning that the spaces are larger in the upper laminae (and thus, probably, that the permeability is greater). However, it could also be alleged to indicate, in a homogeneous system, a large concentration gradient and therefore a small diffusion coefficient! In view of the other evidence this is unlikely.

There is no evidence for the existence of a critical membrane, or extracellular barrier, at the base of the stratum corneum. If such existed, one would expect (a) more critical change of permeability with stripping, and (b) a definite relation of penetrant solubility to permeability, since the barrier would be provided by activation energy and not bulk diffusion resistance (p. 44). The gradual recovery of impermeability after stripping experiments (Monash and Blank, 1958) is also inconsistent with this hypothesis.

Diffusional Resistance of the Cellular Components

There are two possible routes for a penetrant to traverse in the stratum corneum: through the cells and along the intercellular channels. The former contains all three components of the tissue, the latter only the intercellular substance. The intercellular channels present approx. 0·4% of the total cross-sectional area of the surface (calculated as 400 Å channels on a hexagonal 25 μ lattice) and are longer than the thickness of the stratum because of the extensive interdigitation of the cells. If they were as permeable as fluid they could account for the observed permeability on their own: a total path length of 250 μ in a 50 μ slab, over 0·4% of the area, with a diffusivity of, say, 10^{-3}cm^2/min (a normal value for an aqueous solute; Hodgman, 1963), would give a permeability constant of 160 μcm/min, less than that for dissolved

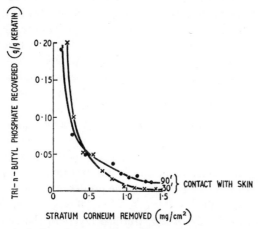

Fig. 17. The mass of tributyl phosphate associated with particles of the stratum corneum which were removed by successive strippings of the skin with adhesive tape after the organic liquid had been in contact with the flexor surface of the forearm for 30 or 90 min.

gases (Table VI) but greater than that for all other substances (Table III). Thus either the intra- or intercellular route could theoretically account for the permeability.

Intensive treatment of skin with polar solvents, but not non-polar solvents, will increase its permeability (p. 20). This might indicate removal of the inter-cellular substance, but might equally well result from a change within the cells, since the keratin spacing is known to change on extraction (Swanbeck, 1959). The same argument applies to the action of detergents, which is in any case equivocal. The penetration of skin by ions and other practically fat-insoluble materials (Table III) shows that some pathway not requiring passage through fat is available; again, however, there is no certainty that the channels are completely filled with lipid. The action of keratolytics on permeability might be taken to show that the keratin is the main barrier within the cells, but as it is also the main mechanical strength of the tissue (Chapter 3) its loss is likely to widen the intercellular channels. The same argument can be applied to the increase of permeability during hydration of the system (p. 17); the keratin undoubtedly swells in a manner peculiar to polar solvents of low molecular weight (Speakman, 1955), but it also weakens the entire structure (Higuchi and Tillman, 1961). Solvent and keratolytic actions therefore do not settle the issue.

In order to study this problem further, it would be desirable to resynthesize the diffusional resistance of the structure from its components. We have made two attempts at this, both unsuccessful; they are recorded here to save repetition of the methods by others. In the first, squamous cells were separated from one another by removing them from the skin surface on adhesive tape, soaking them off in petroleum ether and selecting the slowly sedimenting fractions. They were then allowed to settle and dry. On the addition of water they formed a strong, translucent membrane, flexible when hydrated and brittle when dried. In the second, keratinous polypeptides were extracted from defatted wool by digestion in sodium sulphide and solubilization in sodium dodecyl sulphate. After filtration and de-ionization the solution was dried on to glass. When soaked in hydrogen peroxide a membrane lifted off the glass and could be stabilized in saturated magnesium sulphate. These membranes were weaker than the cellular membranes. Unfortunately both the cellular and keratin membranes were much more permeable to water and alkyl phosphate than skin, so that they had to be discarded as model systems. Nevertheless, theoretically this remains the proper approach.

On the other hand, it is possible in a variety of ways to obtain impermeable membranes composed only of the stratified layers of the epidermis, as was described in a previous section (p. 21). Since these membranes have no "backing material" to affect their properties, they are preferable to skin in studying the cellular components of the stratified layers, though much more difficult to manipulate. These membranes usually have a permeability approximately equal to or rather higher than human skin (Marzulli, 1962; Bettley, 1963; cf. Blank and Gould, 1959, quoted in Table IIIB). The permeability is the same whether or not hair follicles are included in the membrane; we have examined this point directly by the use of a diffusion cell employing very small areas of membrane (Fig. 1B). The permeability is also independent of whether the membrane has been washed in petroleum ether (Table X). In preliminary experiments we have also noted only small changes on washing the under-surface of the membrane with alcohol or 20% acetone. Sodium sulphide solutions, however, greatly raises the permeability and causes visible Brownian motion within the cells, and Bettley and Donoghue (1960) showed that soap solution reversibly increased the permeability of similar membranes to water.

These membrane experiments are no more conclusive than their counter-parts performed on whole skin in determining which component of, or path in the keratinized cell layer determines the whole structure's diffusional resistance, but they do confirm that the material goes through the epidermis rather than the hair follicles, and that a non-polar solvent has little effect on the structure's permeability. This approach is clearly capable of great amplification, and is the most hopeful line in the functional analysis of the tissue.

TABLE X. *The permeability of separated membranes of keratinized cells formed on fish glue tape (A) or rubber latex tape (B)*

Penetrant	Permeability constant (μcm/min) through	
	A	B
Water	160	270
	(68–310)	(60–360)
Ethyl phosphate in water	34	37
	(10–120)	(8–160)
Ethyl phosphate alone	—	2·1

CONCLUSIONS

The highly unspecific barrier resistant to a large variety of chemical insults, demonstrated by the empirical study of skin permeability, is a component of the mature stratified epidermis, the stratum corneum. This system consists of a set of horny plates, bonded together at short intervals and closely interlocked at their edges, so that the channels between them are both narrow and tortuous. The actual route of penetration through this structure remains unknown.

APPLICATION OF DIFFUSION THEORIES TO SKIN PERMEABILITY

Many substances pass through skin at a rate proportional to the concentration difference across the skin (p. 17); i.e. they obey the simplest law of diffusion, that movement is proportional to the driving force, the concentration gradient. The passive diffusion theory may therefore be applied to skin permeability. This theory has been greatly elaborated to account for the behaviour of the very diverse systems which obey Fick's law, and the first thing to decide is which branches of the subject are applicable to the particular problem of skin permeability.

VARIATION OF CONCENTRATION WITH TIME

The basic instantaneous equation of passive diffusion in one direction in a system of constant diffusivity D is:

$$\left(\frac{\partial C}{\partial t}\right)_x = D\left(\frac{\partial^2 C}{\partial x^2}\right)_t \tag{2}$$

where C = concentration of diffusing material.

In words this means that the rate of change of concentration at a point with time is proportional to the curvature of the concentration gradient; if the concentration gradient is linear, the concentration at a point is constant.

This equation can be integrated for given boundary conditions (e.g. $C = C_0$ at $x = 0$, $C = 0$ at $x = l$ for $t \geqslant 0$, $C = 0$ at all points for $t < 0$). Two forms of the solution arise, one suitable for use at times short relative to the equilibration time, and one for use near equilibrium (Crank, 1956). The first form is often used for measuring the movement of a substance into the surface of a thick object, e.g. diffusion into crystals (Barrer, 1951). Such solutions, although they sometimes appear complex, are easy enough to use because they are exact. This is the "simple" theory of diffusion, in which penetrant and penetrated phase do not interact.

In some cases the penetrant interacts with the material through which it moves, so that D is dependent on C. The resultant mathematics is formidable (Crank, 1956), but many attempts have been made to solve particular problems especially in the field of rubber and plastics; e.g. Crank and Park (1949) and Crank (1955) on the movement of chloroform into polystyrene presented on iterative approach. The conceptual basis of relative movement of penetrant and penetrated phase, a matter of importance when polymers swell or when solutions intermix, is still in dispute (Hartley and Crank, 1949; Bearman, 1961).

The main mass of data on skin permeability are concerned only with the steady dynamic state, when the concentration gradient is constant and the rates of movement are constant; under these circumstances both sides of equation 2 are zero, and this part of diffusion theory is irrelevant.

A few data on the change of concentration with time are available, however, and may be considered relative to the "simple theory" in which the diffusivity of the membrane is unaffected by the presence of the penetrant. The delay period (t_d; defined as in Fig. 2, p. 6) for penetration after application gives a measure of the capacity of the membrane for the penetrant, the amount of penetrant held in the membrane at dynamic equilibrium. If the whole stratum corneum were of uniform diffusivity (i.e. a uniform slab) then the capacity l would be

$$l = 6\,pt_d \tag{3}$$

See Appendix I for derivation. Now this product has been obtained in a few cases (Table IV). It is considerably less than the thickness of the presumptive impermeable structure, the stratum corneum, although as it is very easy to underestimate t_d (p. 11) the product may be in error. With this proviso, the results indicate *either* that the material passes through a minor part of the structure (and therefore the capacity is low) *or* that only a small part of the total thickness is a barrier, i.e. the upper layers are comparatively permeable (p. 33). The theoretical treatment can be adjusted to take account of a known relation between diffusivity and depth within the tissue; however, what is required at the moment is far more accurate measurements of the time relations in reaching dynamic equilibrium. This is a promising line.

When the applied penetrant phase changes the diffusivity of the membrane, as water does (p. 17), the "simple theory" no longer applies. This is a very usual case; an extreme example is provided by "saran wrap" therapy (Vickers, 1964) in which corticosteroids are virtually frozen into the membrane by its dehydration. As the theory of "swelling diffusion" is in dispute, it is not profitable to attempt to use the theory on such a heterogeneous system and with such limited data.

DYNAMIC EQUILIBRIUM

The above description applies to the time during which the concentration of penetrant within the membrane is changing. Once a steady state has been built up, the mathematical problem becomes trivial; in equation 2:

$$\left(\frac{\partial C}{\partial t}\right)_x = 0$$

$$\therefore \left(\frac{\partial^2 C}{\partial x^2}\right)_t = 0$$

$$\therefore \frac{dC}{dx} = \text{constant}$$

In terms of the whole membrane thickness, the rate of transfer per unit area, dq/dt is given by

$$\frac{dq}{dt} = p(C_1 - C_2) \tag{4}$$

where p is the permeability constant and C_1, C_2 are the concentrations above and below the membrane. This is equivalent to equation 1 (p. 7) when $C_2 = 0$.

Most of the data available concern the steady state, and can be turned into permeability constants (p. 8). The interpretation of this parameter is therefore the main intent of theoretical descriptions of skin permeability.

Single-phase Membranes

The simplest model on which to interpret the permeability constant is a single phase of high diffusional resistance. The mathematics of the time-relations in reaching equilibrium for such a system are shown in Appendix I. At dynamic equilibrium this equation becomes

$$\frac{dq}{dt} = \frac{D(K_1 C_1 - K_2 C_2)}{h} \tag{5}$$

where K_1, K_2 = partition coefficients between solution and membrane
D = Diffusivity
C_1, C_2 = Concentrations in solutions outside the membrane
h = Thickness of membrane

Interpretation of the partition coefficients

The term K has the same meaning as in bulk phase separations if and only if the thickness of the membrane is large relative to the mean free path of the penetrating molecules; otherwise the distribution will not be that for a semi-infinite backing to the surface. This is certainly correct for the stratum corneum as a whole (20–50 μ thick) or the contents of a single cell (0·5 μ thick) but not necessarily for membranes within the cellular shell or cement (up to 400 Å thick).

Considering only the partition of the penetrant between the stratum corneum and the vehicle in which the penetrant is applied, there is reason to expect K_1 to vary widely for different solvents, depending on their affinity for the solute. Sometimes wide variations of permeability with solvent do occur (Table VII) but often they are surprisingly small. This leads to the supposition that some organic solvents permeate the stratum corneum sufficiently to act as the continuous membrane phase itself, i.e. $K_1 = 1$ for all such liquids.

The partition between the membrane and the underlying solution is, at least in theory, not important, since theoretically $C_2 = 0$ and all molecules reaching the underside of the membrane are rapidly removed. This is not always so in practice, as has been discussed above (p. 14).

Under these assumptions, and only then,

$$p = \frac{K_1 D}{h} \tag{6a}$$

If $K_1 = 1$

$$p = \frac{D}{h} \tag{6b}$$

Interpretation of the diffusivity

The diffusivity or diffusion coefficient, D, is a measure of the resistance to movement of the penetrant molecules within the membrane. Many models have been used to interpret it. The simplest is to assume that the membrane consists of a set of pores, filled with the solution applied to its surface, and is otherwise impermeable.

Porous membrane model

The ratio of the diffusion coefficient through a porous membrane to that in open solution (D_0) is the effective pore area (A_p):

$$A_p = \frac{D}{D_0} \tag{7}$$

This is, on a purely mechanical ("billiard ball") model, related in turn to the relative radii of the molecule (a) and pore (r):

$$A_p = \frac{(1-a/r)^2}{1+2\cdot4a/r} \qquad \text{(8: Pappenheimer, 1953)}$$

The molecular radius referred to is that derived from diffusion in solution by the Einstein–Stokes formula.

This model predicts a large variation of permeability with molecular size even when the "spaces" through which the molecules travel are much larger than the molecules themselves. The model has two similarities with the stratum corneum. Firstly, in practice the applied solution often appears to penetrate the membrane and thus becomes the phase for penetration, as in the model. Secondly, the X-ray and electron-microscope picture of the keratin is one of fibres and "spaces". However, the permeability constants observed do not show a definite critical molecular size above which penetration ceases (p. 8). Since even very large molecules will penetrate slightly there must be a few very large pores. Further measurements of permeability to molecules in the range 1 000–100 000 mol. wt. are required to know whether these are isolated "faults", alongside an otherwise definite porous system, or are the end of a whole spectrum of pore sizes. If the former, the model is useful, for the pores should have a structural meaning. If the latter, it is not.

The pore size of hair keratin has been estimated from the effect of solvents on hair rigidity (Higuchi and Tillmann, 1961). This indicates that no higher alcohols than methanol can get between the fibrils of a keratin matrix. However, higher alcohols do penetrate skin, and more rapidly than methanol (Blank and Scheuplein, 1964). On the face of it, this indicates that transfer through skin is around the cells.

This is probably the most fruitful, and certainly the simplest, of the diffusional models which may be applied to skin.

Viscous flow model

A second model is the frictional system. This concept was devised as part of a formal theory of movement under hydrostatic force, electrical potential

C*

difference, and concentration gradient; the subject is known as the "thermo-dynamics of irreversible processes", and its postulates are lucidly described by Staverman (1954). It describes resistance to movement in terms of frictional coefficients between solute and itself, vehicle and membrane (f_{ss}, f_{sv}, f_{sm}). In dilute solution f_{ss} is negligible, and the relation of diffusivity (D) to frictional coefficients is:

$$\frac{D}{D_0} = \frac{1}{1 + \dfrac{f_{sm}}{f_{sv}}} \tag{9}$$

where D_0 = diffusivity in free solution (Kedem and Katchalsky, 1961).

The terminology, as in all formal thermodynamic theory, is intended as a convenient way of formulating data so that interactions between different forces and movements of different molecular species can be related. At the moment there are insufficient data on such interactions in skin for the theory to be employed, although the means exist for collecting such data.

This model has been used by Blank and Scheuplein (1964) to interpret their skin permeability measurements. They used the formula

$$p = \frac{KRT(C_1 - C_2)}{h(f_{sm} + f_{sv})} \tag{10}$$

where $K = K_1 = K_2$ (i.e. the same solvent above and below the membrane). This equation may be derived from equation 9 on the definition of frictional coefficient in free solution ($f_{sv} = RT/D_0$; Kedem and Katchalsky, 1961). As the value of K remains uncertain so does that of f_{sm}.

The relation between this model and the previous one may be seen by equating (7) and (9)

$$A_p = \frac{K}{1 + \dfrac{f_{sm}}{f_{sv}}} \tag{11}$$

The frictional coefficients, however, imply movement in a continuous medium, rather than movement through pores. They are a measure of the viscosity of this continuous medium. This could be a useful concept in considering different states of swelling of the membrane, during hydration; it would account for continuous variations with swelling better than the pore theory.

This form of theory has been used with great effect in the study of movement in and through polymeric resin beds such as Sephadex, under the influence of hydrostatic, electrical and diffusional fields (Teorell, 1964).

Kinetic theory

The kinetic theory of molecular movement in solution has been developed by physical chemists.

From elementary kinetic theory:

$$D = \lambda^2/2\tau$$
$$= \lambda^2 k \qquad \text{(Tuwiner, 1962)}$$

where λ = mean free path of the molecule
τ = "jump time", interval between movements
k = reaction time constant, i.e. inverse to τ.

The reaction time constant can be described in terms of the heat of activation (ΔH) necessary for the diffusional "jump" and the accompanying entropy change (S)

$$k = \frac{RT}{Nh} e^{S/R} e^{-\Delta H/RT} \qquad \text{(Tuwiner, 1962)}$$

where N = Avogadro's number
h = Planck's constant

$$\therefore D = \frac{\lambda^2 RT}{Nh} e^{S/R} e^{-\Delta H/RT} \qquad (12)$$

In solution the entropy change often dominates the energy change. The extreme case is self-diffusion, seen by the movement of a labelled molecular species through unlabelled similar molecules when $\Delta H = 0$. In membranes, however, one may expect higher values of ΔH, and S may become negligible (Tuwiner, 1962).

If K is known the variation of D with temperature may be deduced from the values of p at different temperatures, since from equation 12:

$$\frac{d(\ln D)}{dT} = \frac{1}{T} + \frac{\Delta H}{RT^2} \qquad (13)$$

However, K is, in general, unknown. If we make the assumption that $K = 1$, i.e. that diffusion is in the applied phase, a Q_{10} of 1·4–3 at 300° K gives values of ΔH between 6 and 20 kcal/mole. This is only true if the membrane is homogeneous, otherwise pore widening or fibre parting with temperature rise will cause a change in p, quite unrelated to the molecular jump within the diffusing phase. Thus "heats of activation" derived from measurements of skin permeability at different temperature (e.g. Blank and Scheuplein, 1964) must be treated with reserve: they do not necessarily describe the energy of activation within the diffusing phase.

Multiphase Membranes

Movement through a multiphase system is normally visualized as a sequence of diffusions through single phases; equilibration at the interphase boundaries is considered to be complete. Mathematical description of the steady state in such a set is straightforward (e.g. Tuwiner, 1962), and the unsteady solution is also possible, although the mathematical formulation often appears forbidding (e.g. Higuchi, 1960).

One concept which has been applied to the skin is that of two thin lipoidal membranes each of permeability constant $2p$ separating a well-mixed reservoir aqueous phase of thickness l (Treherne, 1956). For this system

$$q = p(t - t_d(1 - e^{-t/t_d}))(C_1 - C_2)$$

and
$$l = 4pt_d \qquad\qquad \text{(15; Appendix IB)}$$

where these symbols have the same meaning as before.

Such models can be constructed to fit any observed structure, or to fit any observed relation between permeability and molecular characteristics. Treherne's model accounts for the delay period (p. 6) in terms of equation 15. As is shown in Appendix I, other models will produce a similar delay period; indeed any "thick" membrane must have a delay period. Treherne's model also accounts for the relation of permeability to ether: water partition coefficient which he had observed. However, later workers have found that purely water-soluble penetrants pass through skin quite rapidly (Table III), so that it is unlikely that effectively complete lipoidal membranes occur in the stratum corneum. (They do, however, over the cornea; Maurice and Mishima, 1961).

When one of the phases of a multiphase system becomes very thin (an "interphase"), it is only the movement into or out of it that matters, i.e. D becomes irrelevant, and K all-important. The cell membrane is such a case, which has generated an enormous mass of data and theory. The movement across an interphase is controlled by the energy required for a molecule to enter it. For an uncharged interphase this can be measured by the relative solubility of the molecule in the solution and the interphase material in bulk (i.e. K, although in a thin membrane the distribution may not exactly follow the bulk partition since one phase is not semi-infinite in extent). The mathematics of such systems has been described by Davson and Danielli (1952).

If the interphase is charged, only neutral molecules or molecules of unlike sign can diffuse through it readily. The application of charged models to passive ionic movements in cells is currently of great interest (e.g. Passow, 1964). Beament (1961a) has shown that a charged lipid layer on the surface of cockroach cuticle is responsible for its ability to absorb water (Beament, 1961b).

If there is a continuous layer around each of the horny cells of the stratum corneum, then similar considerations, and mathematics, may be applicable to the stratum corneum.

CONCLUSIONS

Many penetrants appear to penetrate in the phase in which they are applied, otherwise the partition coefficient between vehicle applied and water would have a larger effect on the permeability. The pore size of the structure through which they move appears to have a continuous gradation. Either these "pores" open with increased temperature or the process of travel through them requires considerably more than the normal thermal energy of a molecule. Viewed in an alternative manner, the friction between membrane and diffusant rises steeply with molecular size, and falls sharply with a rise in temperature.

The few penetrants which have been tested appear to fill only a small fraction of the barrier system.

None of these theoretical points enables one to decide which component of the tissue is the diffusional barrier. The absolute values of permeability constant observed empirically can be used to determine D for the various components only when such a decision has been taken. Thus if penetration is through the cells, the partition coefficient is unity and the keratin is the diffusional barrier, then for water:

$$D = ph \qquad\qquad (6b; \text{ assumes } K = 1)$$
$$= 2 \times 10^{-9} \text{ cm}^2/\text{sec}$$
$$(p_{H_2O} = 10^{-6} \text{ cm/sec, Table III}; h = 50 \ \mu)$$

on Pappenheimer's model, the available area is then

$$A_p = \frac{D}{D_0} \qquad\qquad (7)$$
$$= 2 \times 10^{-4}$$
$$(D_0 = 10^{-5} \text{ cm}^2/\text{sec}; \text{ Hodgman, 1963})$$

i.e. 1/5 000th of the area is available for penetration.

Since the permeability constants for other penetrants are mostly much less than that for water, while the diffusivity in free solution of molecules varies only as $M^{\frac{1}{2}}$, A_p for other molecules is a lot less than 1/2 000. This fits in with the work on wool (p. 41).

Alternatively, if the shells of the keratinized cells are the diffusional barriers they must be an order of magnitude more impermeable since they are only one-tenth as thick (i.e. $A_p \leqslant 2 \times 10^{-5}$).

Finally, if one assumes that the cells are even more impermeable than this and that penetration is actually via the intercellular channels, then one may calculate the diffusivity of the intercellular substance. Thus, if $K = 1$ and the interdigitation of the cells results in a path length $5 \times$ the thickness of the membrane, $h' = 250 \mu$. Also, there is one 400 Å channel around each 25μ cell, i.e. approx. 0.4% of the cross-sectional area of the membrane is channel. Then, for water

$$D = \frac{ph'}{A'} \quad (A' = \text{fraction of area which is channel}).$$

$$= 2 \times 10^{-6} \, \text{cm}^2/\text{sec}$$

Thus, if diffusivity of a penetrant through the intercellular material was 10–20% of its diffusivity in water, this would account for skin permeability. Such values do not appear inherently unlikely from the structure of the intercellular channels. Only gases penetrate skin too rapidly to be accounted for by this route.

ACTIVE TRANSPORT

There is some evidence that water is actively transported into the skin. Folk and Peary (1951) found continued uptake of water by covered human feet. Buettner (1953, 1959a, b) placed saturated solutions of known vapour pressure in closed containers over the forearms of subjects, and found that the containers lost weight when the solution vapour pressure exceeded a certain value; at first he believed the critical vapour pressure, which he termed neutral relative humidity, to be 26 mm Hg (approx. 50% s.v.p. at skin temperature) but in his later papers he amended this figure to 35 mm Hg ("85% neutral relative humidity").

Buettner's methods have been criticized on two grounds: firstly, that he did not wait long enough to reach equilibrium between the water vapour and the stratum corneum, so that the inward movement was just into the stratum corneum, and, secondly, that there was sufficient water loss around the margin of his skin cup to account for the water "intake" from the solution. In his later work Buettner continued his experiments for several hours so as to answer the first criticism.

Dirnhuber and Tregear (1960) performed a similar experiment, in which the vapour pressure within a small enclosed container over the skin forearm was measured by the dew-point on a polished surface (Fig. 18). After enclosure the aqueous vapour pressure rose exponentially to a value less than the saturation vapour pressure at the skin temperature (Fig. 19) and then rose much more slowly. After 4 h it had not reached the saturation vapour pressure, and even when it was artificially raised by drawing water on to the hygrometer and then vaporizing it, it fell again thereafter (Fig. 19). Thus the equilibrium vapour pressure at this time after enclosure was, as Buettner predicted, less than the saturation value, by 3–5 mm Hg. Since the flow of water through the skin was approx. 0·2 μg/cm²min mm Hg (as calculated from the exponential phase of vapour pressure rise), the experiments indicated

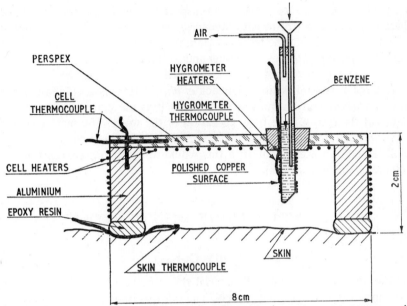

FIG. 18. Heated container with hygrometer, for measuring water vapour pressure rise over skin.

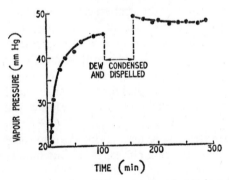

FIG. 19. The vapour pressure rise within an enclosed container (Fig. 18) on a man's back. The container was heated to 3° C above the skin surface temperature except in the interval 120–180 min when it was allowed to cool.

an inward transport, or sideways leak of 0·6–1·0 μg/cm² min. This is small relative to the total mass of water necessary to equilibrate the stratum corneum with water vapour of high relative humidity: Blank (1952) showed that at 90% relative humidity keratin takes up nearly its own weight of water, i.e. approx. 5 000 μg/cm^2 skin. Thus either of the theoretical objections given above is valid: the system may still have been taking up water in the keratin, or may have been leaking around the edge, in both Buettner's and our experiments. The active transport of water remains unproven.

There is no evidence for active transport of ions in mammalian skin as there is in frog skin (for recent references, see Takenaka, 1963). The amount of potassium and chloride removed from the skin surface by washing after a week's insensible water loss, sweating and washing both having been avoided, was very much less than the mass calculated from the insensible water loss, considered as isotonic saline (Hancock *et al.*, 1929). This could, however, be due to a passive inward movement of the salt as the saline became concentrated at the skin surface by evaporation of the water. The mass recovered was equivalent to approx. 10^{-4} meq. KCl/cm^2 (2 meq. over the whole body). If distributed in a depth of 10 μ this would amount to a concentration of 100 meq./l, i.e. near isotonicity.

PRACTICAL CASES OF SKIN PENETRATION

LOSS OF BODY CONSTITUENTS

The only serious losses of material through the skin surface of a non-sweating man are water and protein. The salt loss is 10–20 mg KCl/day with negligible sodium loss (Hancock *et al.*, 1929). The keratinous cells of the skin surface are gradually lost, at a rate dependent on the amount of rubbing they receive. The turnover time for the stratum corneum in man has been estimated from disappearance of stained layers at 32–36 days (Volkmann, 1950). If the thickness of the stratum corneum is 50 μ this represents a loss of approx. 1·5 μ/day or from the whole body 1·4 g protein/day (0·15 mg/cm^2 of material which is 50% protein from an area of 1·8 m^2). Although this is a significant proportion of the minimal total protein turnover in man (4–7 g/day; Lovatt-Evans, 1945), it is a small rate compared with the loss of water (0·1 μg/cm^2 min, cf. 50 μg/cm^2 min).

The insensible water loss in man is one-third to one-half from the lungs and the rest is through the skin (Jores, 1931; Burch and de Pasquale, 1962). The absolute mass lost is approx. 500 g/day. This is clearly not just a concomitant of desquamation as Rothman (1954) suggested. It is also not all via the sweat glands, for anhydrotics lose as much water as normal people in a cool environment (Richardson, 1926), although some of it may be, for pulses of "insensible" sweat have been detected (Gasselt and Vierhout, 1963). The inward active transport of water discussed in the previous section only amounts to 25 g/day and thus would not have much effect on the insensible water loss.

This cutaneous water loss is important, both in the water balance of a desert animal (Schmidt-Nielsen et al., 1957) and in the thermal balance of animals (Blaxter, 1962). It is reduced when the skin surface temperature falls, or when the air is humid, since it depends linearly upon the difference between s.v.p. of water at the skin surface and the v.p. in the ambient air (Zollner et al., 1955). It is little influenced by wind (see Chapter 5) and is therefore present under fur or clothing, as well as in bare skin.

RESPIRATORY GAS EXCHANGE

The skin is very permeable to gases (Table VI), so that although it is of much lower area than the lungs a measurable fraction of the total respiratory exchange of CO_2 and O_2 takes place across it. Under normal conditions a man loses 60–300 ml CO_2/h percutaneously and gains a similar volume of O_2 (Fitzgerald, 1957). This is 0·3–1·5% of the lung's basal exchange. The weight of the skin (dermis and epidermis) of a man is approx. 5% of his total body weight (2 mm × 1·8 m^2 = 3·6 l) and as adult skin has a much lower metabolic rate than that of the active tissues (Barron et al., 1948) the percutaneous exchange is a large proportion of its total respiration. This is demonstrable directly by the change in colour of static blood in a limb when it is enclosed in oxygen (Goldschmidt et al., 1934) and by the possibility of measuring oxygen tensions within the skin through an electrode applied to the skin surface (Naylor, 1959).

FACTORS AFFECTING THE LOCAL ACTION OF DRUGS

The local action of chemicals applied to the skin surface should theoretically depend upon their relative speed of penetration through the stratum corneum and removal from the dermis by the circulation; these determine the local concentration of the chemical within the epidermis below the barrier layer.

The speed of penetration is dependent upon the concentration of the drug applied (p. 6), and upon the vehicle in which it is applied. The vehicle is usually an ointment, which has two advantages over a liquid solvent apart from any effect on permeability: it is effectively involatile, and may be retained on the skin in greater thickness than a liquid. Both these factors make it a more constant source than a drug in a liquid. Ointments do not appear to enhance penetration; indeed salicylates penetrate slower from ointments than from solvents (Loveday, 1961). As there is evidence (p. 40) that penetrants often cross the stratum corneum in the phase in which they are applied, a highly viscous phase might be expected to penetrate slower.

One other factor concerned in ointments is the permeability of the ointment itself, outside the skin. Many ointments are emulsions, so that if the active ingredient is in the dispersed phase and has a high partition coefficient relative to the continuous phase diffusion through the ointment is slow; the exact mathematics for spheres and spheroid emulsions have been calculated by Higuchi *et al.* (1957). An emulsion's impermeability is only of importance if it exceeds that of the skin, which is only the case when the partition is extreme, or the ointment is very thickly pasted on the skin.

The rate of removal of the drug from the dermis is dependent on the local circulation (p. 14). Thus a vasoconstrictive drug may have a positive feedback action; when sufficient of the drug is present to cause constriction, more can accumulate. In the extreme case, when removal of the drug is negligible, the local accumulation may be calculated from the permeability constant:

$$\frac{dq}{dt} = p(C_1 - C_2) \tag{4}$$

$$= \lambda \frac{dC_2}{dt}$$

where λ = depth of tissue in which the drug (concentration C_2) is distributed.

Hence $$C_2 = C_1(1 - e^{-pt/\lambda}) \tag{16}$$

Since the thickness of the dermis is approx. 0·1 cm and the permeability constants found for small organic molecules have often been in the range 0·1–10 μcm/min the time-constant of this equation is 10^4–10^6 min, or in common-sense terms a day's contact with even a rapidly penetrating drug will only produce a dermal concentration which is a small fraction of that on the surface, and increase of p should linearly increase the dermal concentration achieved.

One practical case which illustrates these points is the dermatological use of steroids. There is evidence that steroids are absorbed percutaneously (Scott and Kalz, 1956; Malkinson 1958, 1960; Goldzieher and Baker, 1960), but it is difficult to obtain therapeutic concentrations in the skin percutaneously. When the area is covered with a water-impermeable layer, better therapy is obtained (Wells, 1957; Goldman and Cohen, 1963; McKenzie and Stoughton, 1962). This can be accounted for as the action of two factors: the permeability of the stratum corneum is increased as it becomes hydrated (Vickers, 1964), and the vasoconstriction induced by the steroid once it reaches the dermis prevents its removal by the circulation.

SYSTEMIC ACTION OF PESTICIDES

The efficiency of the skin as a protective barrier is vividly demonstrated by the paucity of cases of percutaneous poisoning by industrial chemicals; only long-term cumulative poisons are considered hazardous by this route (Snyder, 1960). One of the most toxic cumulative poisons, tri-*o*-cresyl phosphate, is fortunately an extremely poor penetrant (Table III), but even rapidly penetrating organic liquids have to be present for a long time over a large area to introduce large quantities into the system. For instance, a liquid penetrating at 10 $\mu g/cm^2$min over 2 000 cm^2 would still only enter at 20 mg/min. This is roughly equivalent to immersion of both a man's arms in, say, an industrial solvent. Few materials are sufficiently toxic for this rate of intake to matter, but some pesticides are (e.g. the mean lethal dose of dieldrin to rats is 40 mg/kg, and of parathion 3–20 mg/kg; Negherbon, 1959). Thus less than 1 g ingested by a man may cause death and many fatalities have resulted from their use. Parathion is alleged to have poisoned more than 6 000 people in Japan (Namba and Hiraki, 1958) and dieldrin affected a large proportion of the spray workers using it to disinfect dwellings in various tropical areas (Fletcher et al., 1959). Cases of dinitro-o-cresol poisoning (Bidstrup and Payne, 1951) and thallium poisoning (Aman, 1962) have also been reported.

Parathion is a liquid of low, but not negligible volatility (6×10^{-4} mm Hg at 25° C; Negherbon, 1959). The likely evaporation rate from such a liquid in a wind can be calculated on meteorological theory (Pasquill, 1949); in a 1 m/sec wind a small area of parathion should evaporate at approx. 0·1 $\mu g/cm^2$ min. Contamination of skin with liquid can reach a maximum of 1 mg/cm^2 (Taylor, 1961; Kligman, 1963) before it begins to run off, but it is likely that most practical densities of parathion contamination were much less than this; an impaction of 60 mg/h on a spray-man (Durham and Wolffe, 1962) means 600 mg/working day, or 33 $\mu g/cm^2$ on 1·8 m^2. The contamination would thus last at least 5 h, and probably much longer, as the liquid would be held in the keratin rather than on its surface. The permeability of cat skin to parathion is 1·5 $\mu cm/min$, i.e. approx. 1·5 $\mu g/cm^2$ min from the undiluted liquid (Fredriksonn, 1962b). A rate of this magnitude maintained over an appreciable proportion of human body surface for a working day would introduce a probably lethal dose: 1·5 $\mu g/cm^2$ min over 10 000 cm^2 for 500 min = 7·5 g, or 110 mg/kg.

Dieldrin is a solid of negligible volatility. Its toxic action is cumulative (Fletcher et al., 1959). During routine spraying operation Durham et al. (1959) showed that up to 0·1 mg/cm^2 of the material accumulated on exposed areas of the body and suggested that long-continued percutaneous ingestion caused the poisoning. Direct measurement of penetration through excised skin showed an extremely slow penetration rate (Tregear, 1964b). Later experiments showed that a rate ten times as great could be obtained by bathing the undersurface of the excised skin in organic solvents, so that the rate in life may be considerably higher than in the published in vitro experiments. Nevertheless, even the highest rates are extremely slow, so that percutaneous poisoning with dieldrin must be a very prolonged process indeed to be harmful.

In summary, it requires a combination of gross exposure and high toxicity for systemic percutaneous poisoning. With elementary precautions and common sense it is usually possible to banish the risk from pesticides (Durham and Wolffe, 1962).

THE PREVENTION AND REMOVAL OF SKIN CONTAMINATION

Barrier creams or films are often employed to reduce skin penetration by external contaminants (e.g. Towler, 1954; Wells and Lubowe, 1964). These creams provide a phase which has to be filled before penetration through the skin can start and which can be removed, together with the contaminant, without damage to the skin. They thus extend the delay period, and reduce residual entry after decontamination. The mathematics of the effect of emulsive creams has been described by Higuchi *et al.* (1957) and Higuchi (1960). At dynamic equilibrium the effect of barrier creams appears to be slight (Steigleder and Raab, 1962). This is readily understandable, since gels are much more permeable than the stratum corneum. Only if the penetrant has to pass through a continuous phase in which it is barely soluble should its diffusion be greatly decreased (Higuchi *et al.*, 1957).

Removal of skin contaminants is usually accomplished simply by washing, i.e. by removal of excess from the surface (Towler, 1954). In the case of radioactive materials the removal process can be monitored, and Lawson (1964) finds that washing with water usually suffices to remove industrial contamination from nuclear fuel elements. If this, or washing in other solvents, is unsuccessful, the contaminant can be removed practically completely by removing the outer layers of the stratum corneum (Born, 1958; Goldhamer and Carson, 1963).

GENERAL CONCLUSIONS

The outer surface of the skin is an unspecific, rugged, impermeable membrane. It lets no molecule through very readily, but all slightly. Its effectiveness is due to the close packing of the horny plates of which it is formed. Penetration probably occurs through this cornified system, rather than down the hair shafts or sweat glands, but whether through or around the horny plates is unknown. Penetration often appears to be in the phase in which the penetrant is applied, and in this the membrane resembles a porous system rather than an intermediate phase. Penetration only reaches practical proportions when the penetrant is a very small molecule, is present in very high concentration or is highly active, locally or systemically.

CHAPTER 2

Movement of Charged Molecules
The Electrical Properties of Skin

A charged molecule will move under the influence of an electromotive force (e.m.f.) as well as down a concentration gradient. Conduction of electricity through skin is a parallel process to its penetration by ions: it is a measure of the ease of movement of endogenous ions through the least conductive layer. This measure is more restricted than permeability, in that it refers to a limited set of ionized molecules. On the other hand, it is possible to change the e.m.f. very rapidly, unlike the concentration gradient, so that the ionized molecules may be made to oscillate.

It is comparatively simple to detect small currents, so that electrical experiments are technically much easier than skin penetration experiments. The techniques have been available for fifty years and over this period many observers have measured conduction of direct (d.c.) and alternating (a.c.) current through skin. The literature on the subject is scattered, ranging from electrical engineering to psychological journals. The present description is an attempt to relate these varied observations to one another, and to point out the structural and theoretical bases of the electrical behaviour.

PRINCIPLES OF ELECTRICAL MEASUREMENTS

PARAMETERS

If a system is unchanged by the passage of current and does not itself supply energy to the current, then the current through it is proportional to the e.m.f. across it (Ohm's law). This is exactly analogous to Fick's law of diffusion (p. 6).

For a direct current (d.c.):

$$i \propto V$$
$$V = iR_0 \tag{1}$$

where V = voltage, i = current, R_0 = resistance.

For a sinusoidally oscillating current (a.c.) of frequency f:

$$V_m = i_m Z_f \tag{2}$$

where V_m, i_m are the time averages (r.m.s.) of the voltage and current. Z_f is termed the impedance at frequency f.

During the passage of a.c. charge will build up in different parts of the system if there are thin, highly resistive membranes within it. Because of this the current will tend to precede the voltage, i.e. the current maximum will be reached earlier than the voltage maximum. This is termed being out of phase, and is specified by the phase angle (ϕ); if $\phi = 0°$ the voltage and current rise and fall together, if it is $90°$ the current maximum occurs as the voltage is zero. The two parameters, Z and ϕ, completely define an ohmic system's behaviour to a.c.

The system may also be specified in a different, but parallel manner. Suppose that during the passage of a.c. of frequency f, the voltage across the system is V_1 when the current is at its maximum and V_0 when the current is zero, we define two proportionality constants, R_f and X_f, such that:

$$V_1 = i_m R_f$$

$$V_0 = i_m X_f$$

X_f is termed the reactance, R_f the resistance, at frequency f.

Now the root mean square value of the e.m.f., V_m, can be shown to be

$$V_m = \sqrt{V_1^2 + V_0^2}$$

$$\therefore V_m = i_m \sqrt{R_f^2 + X_f^2}$$

$$Z_f = \sqrt{R_f^2 + X_f^2} \tag{3}$$

and also

$$\tan \phi = \frac{X_f}{R_f} \tag{4}$$

Hence the ohmic behaviour at frequency f can be completely specified either by X_f, R_f, or by Z, ϕ. It is important to realize that X_f, R_f refer only to the frequency f, and not to all frequencies.

The behaviour to d.c. is simply a special case of equations 3 and 4: at $f = 0$, $X_f = 0$, $R_f = R_0$, and $\tan \phi_0 = 0$, $Z_0 = R_0$.

The application of these parameters depends upon the validity of Ohm's law, just as the use of permeability constant depends on Fick's law. Both laws really mean that the system remains passive and is itself unaffected by the passage of the molecules through it.

ELECTRODE SYSTEMS

In most electrical experiments on skin current is passed between two electrodes applied to the skin surface. The current therefore flows in at one area of skin, through undefined intervening tissue, and out again at the other skin area (Fig. 20). In order to measure the electrical properties of skin

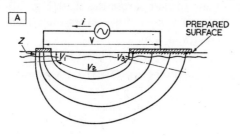

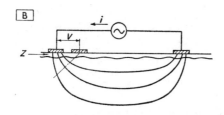

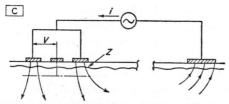

Fig. 20. Arrangements of electrodes for recording the skin impedance (Z), such that $Z = V/i$. Method A is suitable only when $V_1 \gg V_2, V_3$.

it is necessary to know the e.m.f. across one area of skin. In the case of d.c. or a.c. of very low frequency passing through normal skin nearly all the voltage drop is across the skin and not the deep tissue (Barnett, 1938), so that if the voltage across one skin area is made negligible the voltage drop across the other is approximately equal to that across the whole system (Fig. 20A). This can be effected by making one of the electrodes very large and dampening and scarifying the skin with which it is in contact; ECG electrode jelly may be used for this purpose.

When the skin impedance is much reduced the above approximation no longer holds. The skin impedance is reduced by raising the frequency of the applied a.c. At frequencies in excess of 1 kc/s workers have found it necessary to separate the voltage across the skin from the total voltage across the system by the use of a third, non-current carrying, electrode. By appropriate placing of this electrode the voltage between it and the current electrode can be made to approximate to that across the skin (Fig. 20B and C; Barnett, 1938), even when the total voltage drop across the system is largely across the internal tissue (cf. Schwan, 1963).

MEASUREMENTS OF OHMIC PARAMETERS

Direct Current

A galvanometer is a simple, sensitive current-measuring instrument. It is also of low resistance, so that if one is placed in series with skin the a.c. current through the skin can be measured by it, while the voltage across it is small, so that the voltage across the whole system is nearly all across the skin (Fig. 21A). Hence a simple a.c. resistance meter is readily designed (Richter, 1946; Blank and Finesinger, 1946). There is only one proviso: the galvanometer must respond before the net charge through the skin alters the current.

Sinusoidal Alternating Current

If the galvanometer is replaced by a small resistance and the voltage across this measured, e.g. by display on a cathode ray oscilloscope, an exactly parallel a.c. measurement can be made to that of the d.c. instrument. It is necessary, however, to measure two parameters, R_f and X_f (or Z and ϕ). In order to do this it is usual to employ a resistance and capacitance in series with the skin, instead of simply a resistance. The voltage drop across the two impedances is equalized, both in phase and magnitude, and hence the components of the biological impedance are obtained (Fig. 21B).

This method has been employed for thirty-five years (Gildemeister, 1928; Yokota and Fujimori, 1962). Its major drawback is that it is indirect, and therefore time-consuming. However, there are now on the market direct-reading commercial instruments which could be adapted for skin impedance measurements.

Square Wave

A square wave voltage pulse may be viewed as the start of a steady voltage. If it is continued sufficiently long the d.c. resistance is therefore obtained (Fig. 21C; $R_0 = V/i_\infty$), although as the techniques employed are different from the d.c. methods the parameter has usually gained a different name!

The current which flows immediately the voltage is applied is a form of charging current, and is related to the a.c. properties of the tissue: if the wave is really "square", i.e. the rise of voltage is very fast, then the initial current (i_0; Fig. 21C) gives the impedance to a sinusoidal a.c. voltage of very high frequency ($Z_f \to \infty = V/i_0$).

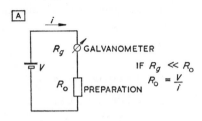

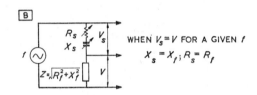

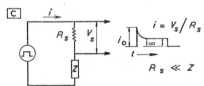

FIG. 21. Three usual methods of measuring skin impedance. (A) d.c.; (B) a.c. half-bridge; (C) square-wave. In the last two methods the voltages are amplified and displayed on an oscilloscope.

CURRENT FLOW THROUGH SKIN

GENERAL FEATURES

When a small e.m.f. is applied across skin, current initially passes very rapidly and then slows down over a period of 0·01–0·1 sec to reach a quasi-steady value. When the e.m.f. is maintained for much longer the current falls further if the current is flowing into the skin (anodal current; Rosendal, 1943) or rises again if it is flowing out of the skin (cathodal current). Throughout this time-course the current is proportional to voltage (Ohm's law) unless the e.m.f. exceeds approx. 2 V, when the current rises rapidly with time whichever way it is flowing and not in proportion to the e.m.f.

The following paragraphs are concerned only with ohmic behaviour uninfluenced by net charge passed, i.e. current flow due to a small oscillating e.m.f. or during the first seconds of a small steady e.m.f. Under these circumstances the terms resistance and reactance, phase angle and impedance are valid.

Skin Resistance and Impedance to Alternating Current of Low Frequency

When a dry metal plate is pressed on to human skin the resistance across the skin beneath it to d.c., and the impedance to a.c. of low frequency (l.f.;

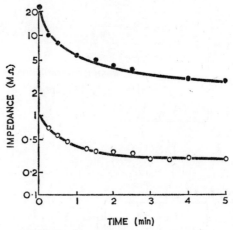

FIG. 22. Impedance of human skin to 1·5 c/s a.c. related to time of contact of a dry silver (●) or agar gel (○) electrode.

1–60 c/s), are both initially very high. They fall rapidly if contact is maintained, and reach fairly steady values after a few minutes; Fig. 22 shows the time-course of the impedance to 1·5 c/s a.c. When a liquid contact is made with skin the resistance, or l.f. impedance, also falls with time (Rosendal, 1943; Blank and Finesinger, 1946; Montagu, 1958) although less than under a dry electrode (Fig. 22). The quasi-steady skin resistance or impedance measured after several minutes' contact time (not current flow) is the parameter referred to in all the subsequent discussion.

This steady resistance is much less under a damp contact than under an initially dry one (Burns, 1950; Fig. 22). The low-frequency impedance is often largely resistive ($\phi < 45°$; $X < R$; Fig. 25), and is highly correlated with, though slightly less than, the d.c. resistance recorded from the same area (Grings, 1953). The two parameters are therefore considered together.

The resistance of human palmar or fingertip skin is less than that of non-sweating arm skin (Table XI). This table shows the very large variation in absolute values between (a) the results of different observers, and (b) within results during one series of experiments. The former may be explained by the considerable variations in technique used, but the latter must indicate a genuine regional variation. In one man Rosendal (1943) found a 100:1

TABLE XI. *Specific resistance and impedance to low frequency of human skin*

Region	Frequency of applied voltage (c/s)	Resistance or impedance (kΩcm^2)	Author
Arm	0 (d.c.)	300– 400	Rosendal (1943)
		100– 700	Krause *et al.* (1953)
		1 000–5 000	Blank and Finesinger (1946)
	1·5	600–1 200	Tregear (1965b)
	10	700	Burns (1950)
Fingertip	0	120	Edelberg *et al.* (1960)
	1	130	Plutchik and Hirsch (1963)
Palm	30	60	Yokota and Fujimori (1962)
	65	80	D. M. Taylor (1961)

TABLE XII. *Specific impedance of saline-dampened skin to* 1·5 *c/s a.c., its reciprocal, the admittance, and the permeability of excised skin to* Na$^+$ *ions in* 0·9 % *NaCl*
For further details see Tregear, 1965b.

Species and region	Impedance (kΩcm^2)	Admittance ($\mu\text{ʊ}$/cm^2)	Permeability (μcm/min)
Man, forearm	880	1·15	—
thigh	—	—	1·1
Pig, flank	12	84	32
Rabbit, flank	18	56	52

variation between the d.c. resistances of different regions of his forearm, although a 5:1 range was more usual. Pig and rabbit skins are much more conductive than human skin (Table XII). Edelberg *et al.* (1960) detected a small variation of skin resistance with temperature, approx. 3% fall per °C rise, equivalent to a Q_{10} of 1·34.

The l.f. impedance or resistance of skin is approximately inversely proportional to the area of contact between it and the conducting solution, paste or metal upon it, i.e. the product of impedance or resistance × area is approximately constant and is termed the "specific impedance" or "specific resistance". Deviations from this relation appear when the area is very small (Fig. 23); under a damp electrode the impedance is less than expected (Fig. 23a; Blank and Finesinger, 1946), while under a dry metal plate it is higher than expected (Fig. 23b). The most likely explanation of these deviations is

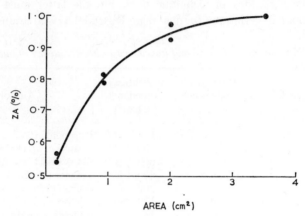

FIG. 23a. Specific impedance (impedance × area) of human forearm skin beneath a 0·9% NaCl: agar gel electrode. Each point represents one observation.

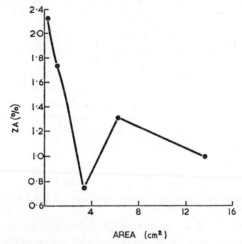

FIG. 23b. Specific impedance of human forearm skin under a dry silver plate pressed on to the skin by 100 g/cm² weight. Measurements were made after 5 min of contact. Each point is the mean of 20 observations.

that water from the damp electrode produces a fringe of conduction through the skin around the edge of the contact area, while under a dry electrode the outer part of the area under the metal is less hydrated than the central part because water escapes from it sideways.

THE IMPEDANCE OF SKIN TO ALTERNATING CURRENT OF HIGHER FREQUENCY

The impedance of skin to a.c. falls as the frequency rises (Fig. 24) and the phase angle (ϕ) rises, i.e. the current flows as through a capacitor. When $\phi = 45°$, the capacitative and resistive currents are equal. At low frequency

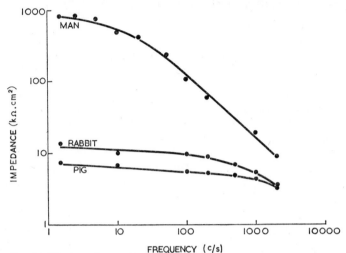

FIG. 24. The impedance of saline-soaked skin related to a.c. frequency.

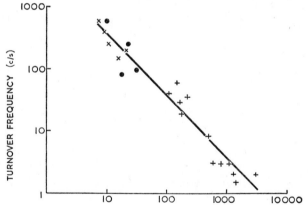

FIG. 25. Relation between frequency at which capacitative current equals resistive current ($\phi = 45°$; "turnover frequency") to impedance at 1·5 c/s a.c., for saline-damped rabbit (●), pig (×) and human (+) skin.

$\phi < 45°$; above a certain frequency, here termed the "turnover" frequency, it rises above 45°, i.e. the capacitative current dominates. The turnover frequency is inversely proportional to the low-frequency impedance (Fig. 25); the proportionality holds good between species.

When the frequency is considerably in excess of the turnover value the phase angle reaches a value that varies little with further increase of frequency (Barnett, 1938; Fig. 28). For human skin the phase angle lies in the range 65–75° over the frequency range 1–15 kc/s (Table XIII).

Over the same frequency range the log of the impedance is linearly related to the log of the frequency (Fig. 24) i.e.

$$Z = kf^{-\alpha} \tag{5}$$

This is to be expected on theoretical grounds, from which also $\alpha = \phi/90°$ (equations 7 and 8, p. 65); calculation of ϕ from α gives good agreement with the directly measured values (Table XIII).

TABLE XIII. *Phase angle (ϕ) of a.c. impedance of human skin, measured directly (tan $\phi = X/R$) or indirectly from the relation of impedance to frequency ($Z = kf^{-\phi/90°}$)*

Author	Frequency range (kc/s)	Phase angle (°)
Direct measurement		
Barnett (1938)	15	71
Rosendal (1944)	2	76
Lawler et al. (1960)	1	75
Plutchik and Hirsch (1963)	1	60
Tregear (unpublished)	1	70
Indirect measurement		
Gildemeister (1928)	0·2–2	68*
Barnett (1938)	2–40	72
Tregear (1965b)	0·5–2	75

* Calculated by Barnett (1938).

In this frequency range the difference between methods of contact with the skin is much less than at low frequency (Burns, 1950). Above 20 kc/s the difference between contact methods becomes even less, the phase angle falls, and the impedance tends to a low, constant value, that of the deep tissue included in this current-carrying path (Yokota and Fujimori, 1962).

THE PATH OF THE CURRENT AND THE SITE OF THE RESISTANCE

PARALLEL PATHS

When skin is pricked (Lewis and Zottermann, 1927), abraded (Rosendal, 1943; Burns, 1950), diamond-polished (Wilcott, 1962) or adhesive tape-stripped (Lawler *et al.*, 1960), both its d.c. resistance and its a.c. impedance fall by an order of magnitude or more, and when a microelectrode wire is forced into the epidermis nearly all of the potential difference due to an external current is found in the outside layers of the skin (Suchi, 1955). Furthermore, an isolated slab of stratum corneum possesses similar a.c. impedance to whole skin (Rosendal, 1945). These experiments show that the epidermal resistance and impedance is near the surface of the skin, i.e. within the stratified layers of the epidermis. They do not prove that the current actually passes through the epidermis; it might pass through the appendages.

When sweat glands are active, most of the current under a dry electrode is due to their activity. Thomas and Korr (1957) showed a linear relation between the current and the number of sweat glands thermally activated in man, and Suchi (1955) showed that the resistance of a fine electrode placed on or near an active sweat gland was much less than that between glands; Edelberg (1964) has confirmed this point. It does not necessarily follow from this that the current actually passes along the sweat gland tube, which is only some 5–10 μ wide (Takagi and Tagawa, 1956) and therefore presents only a minute fraction of the cross-sectional area of the skin. The current may well flow mostly through the epidermis surrounding, and wetted by, the active sweat gland. When the sweat glands are inactive, it is very unlikely that much current passes down them, for the resistance of a microelectrode over an inactive sweat gland pore is no less than that over the intervening epidermis (Suchi, 1955). Thus in a non-sweating area, i.e. most of the human body in a cold or thermoneutral environment, little current is likely to pass down the sweat glands.

On the palm and fingertip the epidermis is up to 10 times as thick as on the general body surface and the sweat glands are more numerous, and are active even at a thermoneutral temperature (Kuno, 1956). Richter *et al.* (1943) showed that palmar and finger skin were approx. 4 times as conductive under a dry electrode as arm skin (cf. also Table XI), and that the region of low resistance expanded and contracted with changes of temperature. Furthermore, Grings (1953) showed that psycho-emotive changes of palmar skin resistance, presumably due to sweat gland activity (p. 70) were proportional to the original resistance values. From these data it appears certain that the sweat glands carry most of the palmar or fingertip current, even while the subject is at rest and in a thermoneutral environment.

There is very little evidence concerning the flow of current down hair follicles. The only direct experiments are those in which silicone grease was used to occlude the hair shafts; this had only a slight effect on the impedance to low frequency a.c. (Tregear, 1965b), and the effect could be duplicated by putting similar grease spots on the epidermis. More experiments would be desirable, but it appears on the present evidence that little current passes down hair follicles.

The much higher conduction through pig and rabbit skin, and its theoretical assessment as a by-pass conduction (p. 66) indicate that much conduction in animals may be via appendages; again, however, more evidence is needed.

LOCALIZATION WITHIN THE STRATUM CORNEUM

The laminae of the stratum corneum can be removed gradually, by stripping with adhesive tape (p. 21). Each stripping reduces the impedance of the

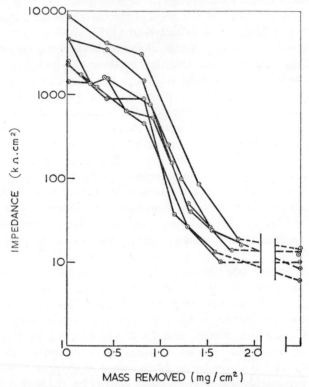

FIG. 26. The impedance of stripped skin to 1·5 c/s a.c., related to the mass of keratin removed from the skin. The broken lines represent the effect of abrasion with sandpaper.

skin, whether measured at 1·5 c/s under a dry metal contact (Fig. 26) or at 1 kc/s, under saline (Lawler *et al.*, 1960). When 1·5–2·0 mg/cm² keratin has been removed the impedance reaches a basal level, little altered by further rough abrasion (Fig. 26). If the mass of keratin removed may be interpreted as depth within the stratum corneum (p. 33), the outermost laminae of the stratum appear to have the highest impedance when dry, but a slightly lower layer within the stratum corneum may have the highest impedance when damp (Lawler *et al.*, 1960). On the logarithmic scale shown in Fig. 26 a discontinuity develops when approx. 1 mg/cm^2 has been removed (20 μ down if half the weight is keratin); this shows that the lower limit of the highly resistive layer is being reached, and not that this depth is particularly resistive (cf. p. 35). Suchi (1955) found a similar discontinuity in the results of his microelectrode insertions approx. 50 μ down in forearm skin and much deeper in palmar skin. The interpretation of his data is more difficult because all the current flow from a needle is not vertical, as it is from a plate electrode, but again his data indicate that the needle had reached the base of the resistive layer, not that it had penetrated a specific barrier layer.

From these data it appears that the impedance of the epidermis lies throughout the stratified layers of the stratum corneum, as does the impermeability (p. 25). Since each are measures of difficulty of molecular movement, one would expect them to give the same answer.

Rosendal (1945) showed that the impedance of powdered keratin was negligible unless it was kept absolutely dry. It follows that the cellular structure of the stratum corneum is essential for its impedance, as it is for its impermeability (p. 36).

THEORETICAL EXPLANATION OF THE SKIN'S OHMIC ELECTRICAL PROPERTIES

GENERAL THEORY

Fricke (1932) produced a theory of electrolytic polarization, i.e. the behaviour of a metal carrying a current immersed in an electrolyte solution. He supposed that passage of a charge across the system provoked a back e.m.f. (V) which decayed as some power (m) of time after the charge had passed

$$V = V_0 t^{-m} \,(0 < m < 1) \tag{6}$$

Hence he related the impedance across the system to the frequency of applied a.c., and found that the phase angle was constant:

$$\phi = (1\text{-}m)\frac{\pi}{2} \tag{7}$$

and that the impedance was inversely related to a power of the frequency (Barnett, 1938):

$$Z = kf^{m-1} \tag{8}$$

Any system in which passage of a current provokes a back voltage which decays as a power function of the time less than unity will follow equations 7 and 8. Such a system is called a "polarization impedance" after the initial physical example, but the occurrence of such an impedance does not imply

D

any chemical reactions within the system. For instance, when a current passes into a system composed of a lot of resistors and capacitors connected in series and parallel, a voltage will be set up across the system which will decay according to the various time-constants of the elements of the system. If there are many elements in the system, the decay may approximate to the power law of equation 6. In that case the system will behave as a polarization impedance, even though no chemical changes have occurred.

Cellular tissues often behave as polarization impedances (Cole, 1932); this is because cell membranes behave as tiny capacitors, and the intercellular channels as resistors connecting them together. When cells are free in suspension the electrical capacity of their cell membranes may be deduced from their polarization impedance (e.g. Pauly, 1962).

THE EQUIVALENT CIRCUIT OF SKIN

The simplest electrical system which adequately mimics the behaviour of skin is a polarization impedance in parallel with one resistance and in series

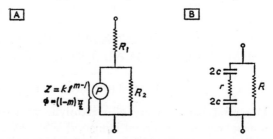

$$Z = k f^{m-1}$$
$$\phi = (1-m)\frac{\pi}{2}$$

FIG. 27. Equivalent circuits of (A) skin and (B) a lamina of the stratum corneum. In B the cell membranes are represented by the two capacitors, the intracellular resistance by r, and the extracellular resistance by R.

with another (Fig. 27; Barnett, 1938). At zero frequency (d.c.) the polarization impedance tends to infinity, and the d.c. current through the system passes through $R_1 + R_2$. At very high frequency the polarization impedance falls to zero, the impedance of the system again becomes purely resistive and equal to R_1. At intermediate frequencies the polarization impedance is greater than R_1 but less than R_2, and so dominates: the phase angle becomes approximately invariant with frequency and the impedance falls regularly with increased frequency.

In human skin R_2 is approx. 100–5 000 kΩcm^2, and in animal skins 10–20 kΩcm^2 (Tables XI and XII). R_1 is the resistance of the deep tissues, and usually lies in the range 0·1–1·0 kΩ; as it is not inversely proportional to contact area it cannot be given in terms of a specific resistance. The polarization impedance is defined by two parameters m and k (equation 8). From the phase angle of human skin in the range 1–10 kc/s (Table XIII), $m \fallingdotseq 0·2$. The parameter k is the impedance of the polarization element at 1 c/s. For human skin it lies in the range 2–10 MΩcm².

It is impossible to make direct estimates of m and k for animal skins, because there are few data (Fig. 24). However, if m is similar to the value for human skin then the inverse proportionality between turnover frequency and low-frequency impedance (Fig. 25) indicates that k also is similar, i.e. that pig and rabbit skins differ from human skin in having a much smaller shunt resistance in parallel with the same polarization impedance.

STRUCTURAL MEANING OF THE EQUIVALENT CIRCUIT

The small series resistance R_1 (Fig. 27) is recorded between electrodes that exclude skin resistance (Barnett, 1938); it is therefore the resistance of deeper tissue.

The large parallel resistance R_2 is a measure of steady conduction through the epidermis and its appendages; its reciprocal is analogous to skin permeability. Over non-sweating general body skin it is probably largely trans-epidermal (p. 22) so that R_2 is a measure of diffusion through the stratum corneum.

The polarization impedance P is an indication that current can oscillate between restraining membranes which restrict its steady passage. The simplest structural explanation of this is that the cells are surrounded by a form of phospholipid membrane (p. 30) and that the d.c. conduction is predominantly around the cells, but it could also be explained in terms of the fibrillar structure of the keratin if the fibrils are surrounded by lipid (p. 31).

A cellular model would provide the set of resistors and capacitors needed to approximate to a theoretical polarization impedance (Fig. 27B). A particular model, designed to simulate the situation in which the outer laminae of the stratum corneum are drier than the inner laminae, is illustrated in Fig. 28. In this system each capacitor is intended to represent one lamina ($r \rightarrow 0$ in Fig. 27B), and the resistance across it the intercellular channels through the lamina. The system behaves similarly to skin under a dry metal contact (Fig. 28), and removal of elements from the model has a similar effect to stripping the skin surface. It should be noted that the model combines R_2 and P of the equivalent circuit (thus illustrating the limitations of equivalent circuits); a pure polarization impedance would have model elements continuing indefinitely in each direction.

As there are 10–100 cell laminae in the human stratum corneum of the general body surface the capacity across each lamina lies in the range 0·1–1 $\mu F/cm^2$.* If this is viewed as the capacity of two cell membranes in series the membrane capacity is 0·2–2 $\mu F/cm^2$. This is similar to that of many live cells (Pauly, 1962). The high phase angle of skin shows that the voltage across

* Deduced from the analogue model of the skin impedance (Fig. 28).

the capacitors decays as a small function of the time. The scant data on animal skin indicating that the polarization impedance is much the same as in human skin agree with the similarity of stratum corneum structure in various species.

In this model the d.c. resistance, R_2, is a measure of the resistivity of the

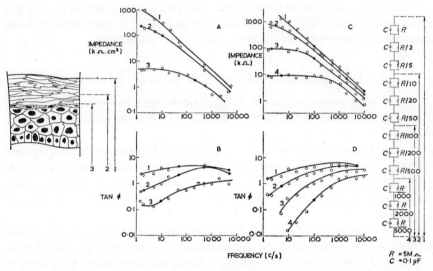

FIG. 28. The impedance and phase angle of human skin under a dry silver electrode (A,B) after various degrees of stripping (see left-hand diagram); and of an electrical circuit (C,D) with successive elements removed (see right-hand diagram).

intercellular channels. If in human skin these are 250 μ long (h') and cover 0·4% of the area of the epidermis (A'; p. 46) then

$$\rho = \frac{R_2 A'}{h'} \tag{9}$$

$$= 0·8–1·6 \times 10^5 \Omega cm$$

This is 1 300–2 600 times the resistance of 0·9% NaCl solution (60Ωcm; Hodgman, 1963).

A similar calculation based on the permeability of human skin to Na$^+$ ions ($p = 1·2$ μcm/min; Table XII) gives

$$D = \frac{ph'}{A'}$$

$$= 6·9 \times 10^{-6} \text{ cm}^2/\text{min}$$

This is 0·8% of the diffusivity of NaCl in aqueous solution ($D_0 = 9·0 \times 10^{-4}$ cm^2/min; Hodgman, 1963). 0·04–0·08% NaCl of this mobility present in the intercellular channels would therefore produce the observed resistance R_2.

The above description is based on the assumption that the d.c. current goes around the cells and the a.c. current goes through them. It does not prove this assumption because of the extreme generality of polarization behaviour; intracellular structure could cause the same phenomena.

NON-LINEAR BEHAVIOUR

NET CHARGE TRANSFER

When a steady current is moved outwards through the skin (cathodal current) the d.c. resistance falls, and vice versa (Fig. 29). Rosendal (1943, 1944) made a detailed study of this phenomenon, and it was also observed by Edelberg *et al.* (1960). The net charge transfer required is of the order of 10^{-3} C/cm^2 (100 μA/cm^2 for 10 sec). The process saturates in that continued charge transfer no longer changes the resistance (Fig. 29). The ratio of the

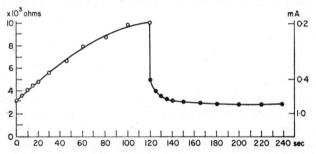

FIG. 29. Time dependence of the resistance at 2 V of 7 cm^2 of skin moistened for 20 min with saturated KCl solution. Ordinates: left, resistance in ohms; right, current in mA. Abscissae: time in sec. ○, Anodic conduction; ●, cathodic conduction. From Rosendal (1943).

two saturation levels of resistance can be as large as 10:1. The a.c. impedance at 1 kc/s is also changed in the same direction, but by a much smaller factor.

Rosendal suggested that these changes were due to ionic depletion in the stratum corneum under an anode, because of a positive charge on the protein which restricted movement of positive ions from the contact solution into the skin; this argument is discussed further below (p. 70).

EXCESS VOLTAGE

A steady e.m.f. in excess of 2 V across the arm skin causes a continuous increase in current, whichever the direction of current through the skin. Coincidentally, pain is felt by the subject and the skin area becomes hyperaemic (Rosendal, 1943). A similar increase of conduction through palmar skin with voltage was observed by Grings (1953), and Cleves and Summer (1962) found a very low "resistance" to 60 V d.c. A 1·5 c/s a.c. voltage also produces non-linearity when its peak value exceeds 1–2 V (Tregear, unpublished observations). As the voltage is increased, the current flow at the voltage peak begins to rise more than proportionally; at this stage no pain is felt. At a slightly higher voltage a "catastrophic event" occurs; the current rises sharply, linearity within the a.c. cycle disappears completely, and the subject feels pain.

The simplest, but unproven, explanation of these events is that above a certain e.m.f. the current is sufficient to move water up into the stratum corneum; this process has been demonstrated directly in excised skin by Rein (1924). This water then carries more current and a whole sequence of changes follows including nerve and sweat gland stimulation.

POTENTIAL DIFFERENCE IN THE ABSENCE OF CURRENT

There is commonly an e.m.f. of 1–10 mV between different regions of skin (Grings, 1953) which varies with time (Fujimori, 1955). Surface abrasion abolishes the e.m.f., i.e. it is transepidermal in origin (Rein, 1926). At least two components of this e.m.f. have been separated. The first is due to diffusion at the skin surface; it is positive outwards, and is largest when a low concentration of electrolyte is applied to the surface (Rein, 1926). The second is an atropine-sensitive negative-outwards potential present after diffusion has been saturated (Keller, 1931).

Rein interpreted the diffusion potential in terms of movement of endogenous ions in a negatively charged protein. The potential could, however, be due to movement of exogenous ions from the contact electrolyte into a positively charged membrane: the negative ions would move in more readily and leave a net positive charge in the contact electrolyte. This is a similar explanation to that offered by Rosendal for his charge transfer results.

USES OF ELECTRICAL MEASUREMENTS

PSYCHO-EMOTIVE SWEATING

Changes in the resistance of, and e.m.f. across, the fingertip or palm skin, may be used to measure the effects of mental stress. The reduction in resistance, produced either by mental stress or by efferent nerve stimulation, has been termed the "exosomatic galvanic skin reflex", the change in e.m.f. the "endosomatic galvanic skin reflex". These names tend to confuse the phenomena with the "galvanic skin reaction" of Ebbecke (1921) which is the change in skin resistance often observed when the skin is subject to local mild trauma.

The galvanic skin reflex can be abolished by peripheral nerve section or ganglionectomy (Richter, 1946) mimicked by sympathetic nerve stimulation

(Richter and Whelan, 1943) and separated from vasomotor changes (Darrow, 1929). It is thus certainly due to sweat gland activity. When damp electrodes are employed, the resistance changes are probably due to events within the sweat glands and ducts themselves; if dry electrodes are used, they may be complicated by epidermal resistance changes when the sweat wets the skin surface.

The changes in e.m.f. across the skin do not exactly parallel the resistance changes (Montagu, 1958). The response to a sudden mental stress falls into two phases, a rapid positive-going deflection which is not accompanied by any resistance change, and a slower negative wave which is related to the resistance change (Takagi and Nakayama, 1958, 1959; Fig. 30). These later

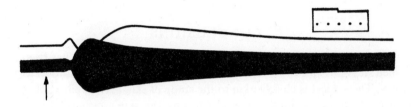

FIG. 30. Simultaneous record of galvanic skin reflex (GSR) and impedance change. GSR was recorded from left thumb. Impedance change was measured between right thumb and forearm with alternating current of 1 000 c/s. Arrow indicates an electric stimulus to the leg. Calibration voltage 1 mV; time mark 1 sec. From Takagi and Nakayama (1959).

events can be abolished by repeated stimuli, leaving the positive wave unimpaired, and the positive wave can also be preferentially recorded if a fine electrode is placed over a sweat pore. Takagi and Nakayama (1959) therefore suggested that the positive wave is a reflection of sweat gland cell activity, while the resistance change and accompanying negative wave are due to rise of sweat in the tube and on to the epidermal surface. Lloyd (1960) also showed that the impedance changes in cat pad skin under a damp electrode paralleled the rise of sweat in the ducts, although Gougerot and Duvelleroy (1960) have criticized his conclusions.

THERMAL SWEATING

The resistance of skin can be used to measure thermal sweating in a limited skin area provided that the electrode used is itself dry and that water is allowed to evaporate from the skin between, or preferably during, the resistance measurement. This may be achieved either by making the contact time short (Thomas and Korr, 1957) or by making the contact area narrow, as in a wire mesh (Rutenfranz and Wenzel, 1958). In order to maintain the relation between resistance and sweat rate it is advisable to force a constant flow of dry air past the sensing element.

EPIDERMAL DAMAGE

The resistance, or impedance to a.c. of low frequencies of damp skin is a measure of its impermeability and hence of the integrity of the stratum corneum. Gougerot (1947) found appreciable changes in the impedance of apparently uninvolved skin around dermatotic lesions. The preceding discussion indicates that the most informative parameter ought to be the impedance to a.c. of very low frequency (approx. 1 c/s) under a well-dampened electrode of at least 1 cm² area. The procedure has not become established as a dermatological diagnostic tool, probably largely because of the unwieldy equipment involved. Commercial electronic equipment is now available that should make such measurements routinely practicable.

CONCLUSIONS

The necessary basic work on the electrical properties of skin has been performed: it is possible to relate empirical data both to structure and to formal theory. The subject is closely akin to the study of skin permeability; electrical measurements are a simple means of testing the skin's permeability to the ions within the stratum corneum.

CHAPTER 3

Force between Molecules
Mechanics of Skin

The mechanical state of the skin *in situ* on the body is complicated to describe or interpret. In some parts of the body the skin is under chronic mild tension, in others it is entirely slack. In some parts it is free to slip over the underlying tissue, and in others it is tightly held. When pulled, skin gives easily until the "slack" has been taken up and is then very difficult to extend. A very large force is needed to tear skin, but if it is maintained taut for a long time it gradually slips. If pressed inwards, skin becomes thinner under the compressing force, with a thicker ridge around the periphery.

Dermatologists have used several tests to assess these properties (Rothman, 1954), but it is difficult to relate them one to another or to interpret the parameters that they measured; the original observers were primarily interested in changes under clinical conditions or treatments. Only experiments in which a known stress is applied and the resultant deformation or strain measured can be interpreted in general terms. There are comparatively few such observations available, but they suffice to show the general outlines of the skin's mechanical behaviour, and allow it to be related to the structure of the dermis which is the major load-bearing tissue in skin.

SKIN EXTENSION: METHODS AND INTERPRETATION

All measurements of skin extension have been performed *in vitro*, in order to measure accurately the stress and strain. Two methods have been used: the extension of a strip of skin and the distension of a circular diaphragm of skin. The excised strips were pulled out by a known weight and the resultant extension measured (Fig. 31, A and B), while a pressure difference was applied across the diaphragms and the resultant curvatures measured (Fig. 31C).

In the strip, or linear, method the stress (T) is the weight (F) divided by the cross-sectional area of the strip

$$T = \frac{F}{A} \tag{1}$$

and the strain (S) is the extension per unit length

$$S = \frac{l}{l_0} - 1 \tag{2}$$

The only difficulty in the strip method is the clamping of the skin. This weakens the adjacent tissue, and makes it necessary to measure extension between two points along the strip (Fig. 31A) or to avoid clamping altogether by obtaining

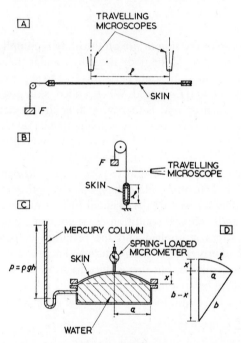

FIG. 31. Methods of measuring skin extension. A, The extension of an excised strip; B, the extension of a band, C, the distension of a diaphragm; D, geometry of C.

a band of tissue from the torso of a small animal or the limb of a large one (Fig. 31B; Harkness and Harkness, 1959b).

The diaphragm method has three advantages: it is easy to measure small distensions, the pressure can be applied and released very quickly, and the tension in the tissue is in all directions parallel to the skin surface instead of in only one direction. Unfortunately, this last point is only true near the centre of the diaphragm; at the edge, where the tissue is clamped, stretch can only be radial. This defect makes it impossible to provide a precise interpretation of the data. The best that can be done is to assume that the edge-effect is negligible, when:

$$T = \frac{pa^2}{4xd}\left(1+\frac{x^2}{a^2}\right) \qquad (3)$$

$$S = \frac{2x^2}{3a^2\,(1+2x^2/a^2)} \qquad (4)$$

(for justification see Appendix II).

If, and only if, stress does not affect the structure of the tissue, one may expect that strain will be proportional to it. This is Hooke's law (in differential form):

$$\frac{dT}{dS} = Y \qquad \text{Young's elastic modulus} \qquad (5)$$

Young's modulus is equivalent to resistivity in electrical conduction, or diffusional resistance in permeability. Its reciprocal, the elastic extensibility (E), is equivalent to conductivity or diffusivity. Hooke's law itself is formally similar to Ohm's law and Fick's law. The main difference in its application is that in a fibrous tissue such as skin it does not apply for small stresses, because a small stress does affect the properties of the tissue: it straightens the fibres out. Once the fibres are taut then further extension is due to elastic stretch within the molecularly arranged fibres, and this may obey Hooke's law, at least approximately, until the tension becomes excessive and the tissue breaks. One further proviso has to be placed on the operation of Hooke's law in connective tissue: maintained tension causes a gradual, irreversible slip, so that for Hooke's law to hold the tension must only be applied for a short time.

The slip under maintained tension is a process dependent on some form of viscous resistance. This process may also obey a linear relationship, provided again that the slip does not appreciably alter the structure:

$$\frac{dS}{dt} = uT \qquad (6)$$

where S is the strain and T the stress, as before, and "u" is a constant, called the "viscous extensibility". Slip can be measured by the same methods that elastic extension is measured, simply by maintaining the tension. It is often found that a tissue slips rapidly at first, presumably due to straightening of fibres, and thereafter obeys equation 6.

ELASTIC EXTENSION

Skin can be stretched reversibly by up to 10–50%, dependent on age and species, provided the tension is not maintained for more than a few seconds.

If the extension is greater, the skin gives way and tears; if the tension is maintained for longer, an irreversible extension is added to the elastic stretch.

The first few per cent of strain are very easily obtained (Fig. 32). The exact quantity of "slack" depends greatly on the initial state of the tissue, and is not

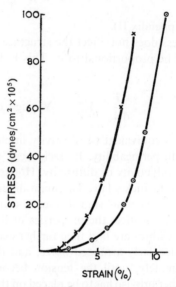

Fig. 32. Extension of excised pig skin at 20° C, as measured by the extension of a strip (×) or the distension of a diaphragm (○).

reproducible. It is present in both the strip and diaphragm methods. Dick (1951) examined the strains in human skin due to small stresses using a diaphragm technique. He found a correlation between the strength at low tension and the elastin content. Unfortunately, he did not calculate the stress he employed (as in equation 3) and so did not produce any absolute values for the skin extensibility.

Once the slack has been taken up, skin behaves very differently. The extensibility becomes small and constant with increasing stress, i.e. Hooke's law holds (Fig. 32), until near the ultimate tensile stress (Rollhauser, 1950). Young's modulus for a given species and age is quite consistent (Rollhauser, 1950; Fry et al., 1962). Where it has been tested, the diaphragm method has yielded similar results to the strip method (Table XIV). Skin is only a little more extensible than tendon, once the slack in it has been taken up. The rodents' skins have the highest extensibility of those tested. The extensibility of human skin falls with age (Table XIV) and female skin is weaker than male skin (Wenzel, 1948). Wenzel also noted that torso skin was less extensible than limb skin, and that the extensibility of an excised strip varied significantly with the direction in which it had been cut from the body. Striae or operation scars greatly reduced the strength found. The few values available of the ultimate tensile stress and strain are shown in Table XV; skin appears to break when stretched by one-sixth to one-half of its original length, but it is not certain how much of this extension is true elastic stretch, and how much is viscous slip due to maintenance of the tension.

TABLE XIV. *Young's modulus (Y) for skin and tendon*
Values quoted are for the strain range of minimal extensibility, when available.

Species and tissue	Y dynes/cm^2 ($\times 10^8$)	Strain range (%)	Author
Rat torso skin	0·8	0–12	Fry *et al.* (1962)
Rabbit back skin	2·1	10–12	Dirnhuber and Tregear (unpublished)
Pig back skin by:			
(a) Strip method	2·6	6–16	
(b) Diaphragm method	2·9	6–11	
Human abdominal skin			
Age (years) 0–6	2·9	10–45	
15–30	6·7	10–30	Rollhauser (1950)
30–50	8·1	10–30	
50–80	11·0	10–30	
Rat Achilles tendon	13	0–30	Burton (1954)
	4	0·3–2	Ciferri *et al.* (1965)
Pig Achilles tendon	7	3–5	Bull (1957)

TABLE XV. *Ultimate tensile stress (U.T.S.) and strain of excised skin*

Species and region	U.T.S. (kg/cm^2)	Strain (%)	Author
Rat back	3*	25	Fry *et al.* (1962)
Rabbit back	7	14	Dirnhuber and Tregear (unpublished)
Human abdomen	50–200	30–47	Rollhauser (1950)

* Calculated from the quoted value in terms of kg/cm^2 collagen.

VISCOUS SLIP

The tendency of skin to slip under continuous tension has been noted many times (e.g. Wenzel, 1948) but has been studied in detail only by Harkness and his collaborators. This group found that rat and chick skin, in common with other connective tissues, extended at a steady rate under a constant tension, after an initial rapid phase (Fig. 33; Harkness and Harkness, 1959a). Except under extreme tension or when the skin had been deliberately weakened, the extension was very slow, and the steady rate was maintained for several hours. The skin broke after it had slipped by approx. 25% of its original length (Fry *et al.*, 1962). The steady velocity of extension was proportional both to the original length and to the stress applied. Thus the linearity between force and effect set out in equation 6 held, and the viscous extensibility (u) could be found. For rat skin $u = 5 \times 10^{-10}$ cm^2/dyne min,

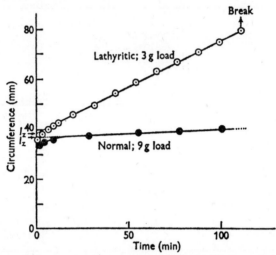

FIG. 33. Effect of constant load on inner circumference of rings of skin from neck of normal and lathyritic chicks. Loading for normal chick 197 g/mm^2 collagen, for lathyritic chick 77 g/mm^2 collagen, calculated for length l_0. (From Fry *et al.*, 1962).

i.e. a force of 2 kg/cm^2 (2×10^6 dynes/cm^2) caused a slip of 0·1% /min. The viscous extensibility of chick, but not rat, skin was greatly increased in lathyrism, the syndrome produced by eating sweet peas (Fry *et al.*, 1962), and the viscous slip of the rat uterine cervix was also greatly increased towards the end of pregnancy (Harkness and Harkness, 1959b). Hyaluronidase had no effect on the viscous slip of skin, but trypsin increased the slip (Harkness and Harkness, 1959a). Wenzel (1948) noted that the viscous slip of human skin was greatly increased over a region containing striae gravidae.

COMPRESSION OR VISCOUS FLOW

Solids and liquids are virtually incompressible; it requires enormous pressure to produce a detectable change in volume (Champion and Davy, 1952). The phenomenon referred to here is compression with a leak, i.e. flow under pressure. It can be observed by pressing a small object into the skin; a depression is formed which does not disappear when the force is removed, but can be massaged away. In order to measure the flow under pressure, one has to apply a known force over a known area, and measure the deformation produced. The main difficulty in doing this is the initial, elastic deformation produced by applying a weight to skin. This is usually large relative to the later, viscous deformation, and as the viscous deformation begins very rapidly it is difficult to disentangle the elastic movement from the early part of the viscous flow. In order to reduce the elastic movement one may choose an area of skin over a hard backing, such as the skin over the shin in man, or a fold of back skin in a rodent (Fig. 34A), and in order to reduce the effect

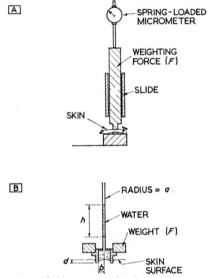

FIG. 34. The measurement of skin compression by the movement of a weighted rod (A) or by displacement within a plethysmograph (B).

the elastic movement one can use a measuring system which responds only to movement of the weight relative to the skin surface, such as the Schade (1912) elastometer, which was later modified and used by Kirk and Kvorning (1949), or a water-filled plethysmographic annulus (Fig. 34B). Although practically attractive, in that measurements can be made simply and rapidly, the plethysmograph has a theoretical flaw: the volumetric displacement is ambiguous. Water will be displaced if the annulus sinks into the skin, but it will also be displaced if the intradermal fluid under the annulus moves into the centre of the ring. If this second process is neglected, the skin deformation under the annulus is

$$d = \frac{ha^2}{b^2} \tag{7}$$

(cf. Fig. 34B for meaning of symbols).

There are very few measurements available of viscous flow in the skin. Earlier workers (Tui *et al.*, 1949; Kirk and Kvorning, 1949) concentrated chiefly on the elastic deformation, and did not clearly define the difference

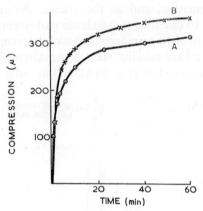

FIG. 35. A, Compression of a fold of rat skin by a weighted rod (radius 0·8 cm; force 910 *g*); B, compression of the theoretical model system (equation 10; $\beta = 1\cdot2$ min $^{-1}$, $h_0 = 400\mu$).

between the two. The results quoted below come almost entirely from a short series of experiments in our laboratory (Tregear and Dirnhuber, 1965).

Viscous flow starts very rapidly, and slows down continuously over the subsequent 100 min (Fig. 35). The relation of deformation to time is not

TABLE XVI. *Maximal compression of skin, excluding elastic component*

Species and region	Compression (mm)	Author
Rat back	0·3	Tregear and Dirnhuber (1965)
Human forearm	0·6	Tregear and Dirnhuber (1965)
Human leg	0·5–0·6	Kirk and Kvorning (1949)
	0·65	Tregear and Dirnhuber (1965)

exponential; there is a long "tail" of continued deformation. The total deformation is in the range 0·3–0·7 mm in human and rat skin (Table XVI). The speed of deformation, but not the total deformation produced, varies greatly with the force applied and the area of contact (Fig. 36). In rat skin hyaluronidase greatly increased the speed of deformation (Fig. 36). The results obtained on rat skin by the plethysmographic method were similar to those obtained by the direct method, despite the theoretical objection to plethysmography.

Day (1949, 1952) measured the flow of an aqueous solution through excised mouse fascia under a small pressure difference. He found that the flow increased by a large factor when hyaluronidase was added to the solution, and decreased again when one of a variety of macromolecules (agar, starch, gelatin) was added afterwards.

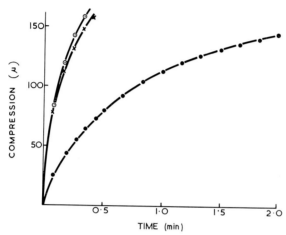

FIG. 36. Compression of a fold of rat skin by a 910 g force acting on a rod of diameter 4 mm (×) or 8 mm, before (●) and after (○) the action of hyaluronidase.

STRUCTURE RESPONSIBLE FOR MECHANICAL PROPERTIES

The elastic modulus of skin is much greater than that of passive muscle (Pryor, 1952) or fat, and is in the same range as the strengths of tendons (Table XIV). The collagen in the connective tissue is therefore almost certainly the main strength of skin. In most species the main connective tissue layer is the dermis (Fig. 37).

Bulk flow of liquid can only occur in an unencapsulated system, so that unless cells are broken or transported bodily flow in tissue must be extra-cellular. The dermis is the main extracellular tissue of skin, and is reduced in thickness on skin compression (Fig. 38) so that viscous flow, like elastic extension, appears to be a property of the dermis.

DERMAL STRUCTURE: FIBROUS PROTEINS

The dermis is bounded on the one hand by the epidermis and on the other by the cutaneous muscle or fat cells (Fig. 37). It is pierced by the hair shafts,

E

which penetrate through most of its thickness (Fig. 37). There are comparatively few cells in the dermis; its main structural component is the collagen (Fig. 39). Collagen represents 75% of the dry weight of human skin

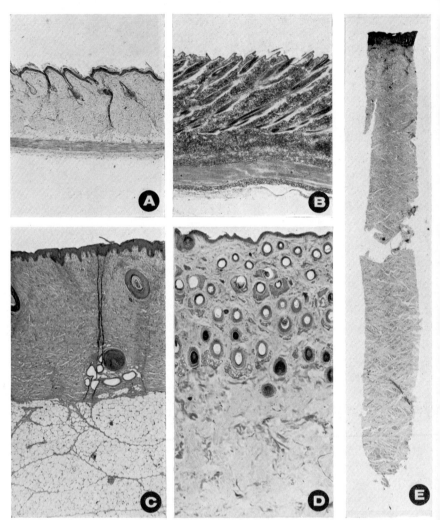

FIG. 37. Low power photomicrograph of flank skin from the rat (A), rabbit (B), pig (C), horse (D) and hippopotamus (E). All sections stained with haematoxylin and eosin. A–D, × 50; E, × 7·4. Note the panniculus carnosus in A and B. (Crown copyright reserved.)

(Neumann and Logan, 1950; Weinstein and Boucek, 1960) and approx. 18–30% of the volume (3–5% nitrogen/g wet weight, Rothman, 1954; 6 g collagen/g nitrogen, Bowes and Kenten, 1949). In young rat skin there is

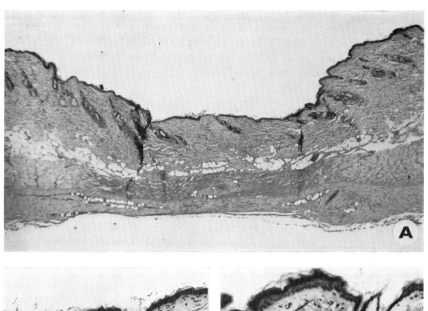

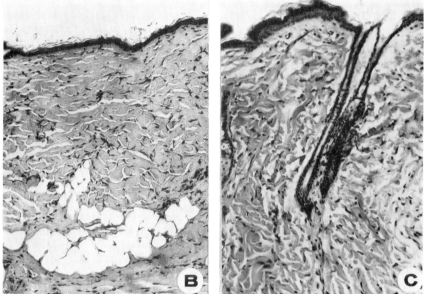

Fig. 38. Rat skin fixed while compressed by a weighted rod. A, Low power micrograph (× 50) of compressed skin and adjacent regions. Note compression of all layers. B, Detail of compressed dermis (× 160); C, detail of dermis from region adjacent to compression (× 160).

E*

less collagen, approx. 10% by volume (g/g wet weight; Smith, 1964). The volume fraction of collagen in skin rises with age, although the absolute mass of collagen per unit area of human skin falls (Harkness, 1964).

Collagen is formed in the spindle-shaped fibroblasts which are found

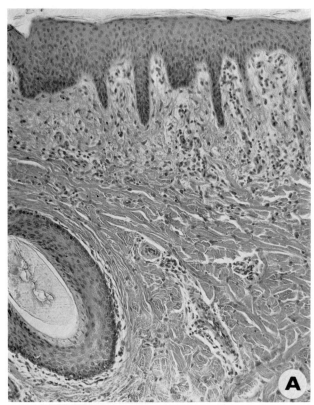

Fig. 39A

Fig. 39. Collagen of the mammalian dermis. A, Pig; B, hippopotamus. Note the finer fibres around the hair and adjacent to the epidermis, and the parallel fibres within the large bands of collagen in hippo skin. van Gieson. × 160. (Crown copyright reserved.)

throughout the dermis (Fig. 39; Montagna, 1962). A triple helix of polypeptide chains is formed within the cell and extruded as the soluble element of the collagen fibre, tropocollagen (Fitton-Jackson, 1953). Tropocollagen molecules line up to form the actual fibrils of collagen, which then grow in size by gradual accretion. Mature collagen fibrils of the dermis are 600–1 400 Å in diameter (Braun-Falco and Rupec, 1964; Gross and Schmitt, 1948).

The internal structure of the mature collagen fibril has been studied in great detail; for a complete review see Harkness (1962, 1964). Each fibril is composed of rows of tropocollagen molecules joined head to tail and arranged in parallel, staggered rows. The tropocollagen molecule is 2 800 Å long, and the characteristic 650 Å bands of collagen (570 Å in skin; Braun-Falco and Rupec, 1964) are due to the staggering of the parallel array. Tropocollagen is

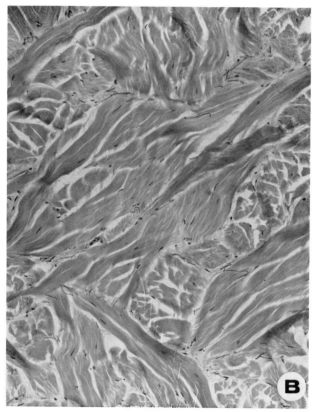

Fig. 39B

itself composed of three polypeptide chains twined in a helix, each of 100 000 M.W. Two of the three chains are identical to one another. When collagen is denatured by heating above 60° C to form gelatin or glue, the tropocollagen molecule itself unwinds; otherwise soluble collagen may be reprecipitated in banded forms, like natural collagen. The polypeptide chains themselves consist of four 25 000 M.W. sub-units connected by ester linkages.

Collagen is unusual among proteins in its large content of proline, hydroxyproline and glycine. The principal links between the polypeptide chains in the triple helix of tropocollagen are the hydrogen bonds between the amine of glycine and the carboxyl of the amino acids. Collagen fibres can be stretched greatly *in vitro*, as seen by the increased separation of their bands (Fig. 41). This degree of stretch is unlikely to be reversible, as the structure of the tropocollagen molecule could not accommodate so large a change (Dickerson, 1964).

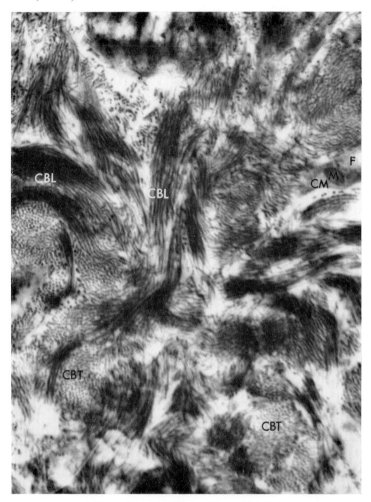

FIG. 40. Typical collagen bundles in the dermis. A small portion of a fibroblast is shown at F, the cell membrane can be distinguished at CM with a mitochondrion above (M). The tip of the process of the fibroblast merges with the collagen bundles (CB). CBL, Collagen fibres cut longitudinally; CBT, collagen bundles sectioned transversely. × 5 500. (From Causey, 1962.)

Collagen fibrils in the dermis are arranged parallel to one another in large sets. Anastamoses between adjacent fibrils occur infrequently, if at all (Braun-Falco and Rupec, 1964). The space between the fibrils is usually similar to,

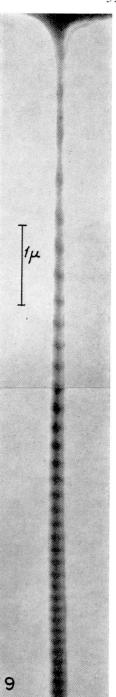

or less than, their diameter. These parallel sets are the collagen fibres of optical microscopy. They are 1–20 μ across, and are often perpendicular to adjacent sets (Fig. 40). Most of the fibres lie parallel to the skin surface, except in very thick skin. It is not known whether these fibres are really separated in life (Jarrett, 1958); the histological picture is highly dependent on the degree of swelling or shrinkage produced by the fixative. The fibrils at the centre of the histological fibres may be in a different environment from those at the periphery, because of the difficulty of diffusion through the fibre (Borysko, 1963); nevertheless, the diameter of fibrils throughout a fibre is remarkably constant.

In old age or under prolonged solar irradiation, the dermal collagen degenerates and the skin becomes slack. Histologically the degenerate collagen resembles elastin, and the effect has been termed senile elastosis, but in the electron microscope the degenerate fibrils may be seen to arise from normal collagen (Banfield and Brindley, 1963; Loewenthal and Pienaar, 1960; Tunbridge et al., 1952). However, this subject is still controversial (Tunbridge, 1964). In other circumstances the fibril structure of collagen is remarkably invariant.

The other two fibre types in the dermis, reticulin and elastin are present in comparatively small amounts. Reticulin fibres make up only 0·4% of the dry weight of human skin (Montagna, 1962). They are fine argyrophil fibres, readily distinguished histologically from collagen (Jacobson, 1953) and distributed particularly around blood vessels and hairs and close to the epidermis. Reticulin fibres stain intensely with periodic acid–Schiff's reagent (Montagna, 1962) and similar fibres from the kidney contain a large proportion of polysaccharide (Kramer and Little, 1953). Despite their distinct location and polysaccharide association, reticulin fibres appear to be composed of collagen fibrils: their amino acid content is the same

FIG. 41. Fibril from rat tendon, enormously stretched by peeling back of collodion supporting film. × 21 000. (From Schmitt et al., 1942.)

as that of collagen (Bowes and Kenten, 1949) and their fibrils have the same cross-banded appearance (Gross, 1950).

Elastin, on the other hand, is a recognizably different protein from collagen containing much less hydroxyproline (Bowes and Kenten, 1949). It represents 4% of the dry weight of human skin (Weinstein and Boucek, 1960), and therefore approx. 1% of the wet weight, or volume. Histologically, elastin appears as branching, twisted fibres (Montagna, 1962). It is amorphous in the electron microscope or under X-ray diffraction analysis, and little is known of its macromolecular structure. A similar protein is found in high concentration in the bovine ligamentum nuchae. This protein is easily and reversibly extensible over a large proportion of its resting length (Bull, 1957); hence it has gained its name.

GROUND SUBSTANCE

The fibrous proteins form 10–30% of the dermis. The rest of the volume is filled by the interfibrillar and interfibre material, termed the ground substance. This material is either a gel or a solution. In addition to the usual crystalloids of extracellular fluid it contains protein and polysaccharide components. The protein is partly soluble collagen ("procollagen"; Harkness, 1962) and probably partly non-collagenous; little is known of the non-collagenous protein. On the other hand, the polysaccharides of the ground substance have been studied intensively.

The two major components in pig and human skin are hyaluronic acid and chondroitin sulphate "B" or dermatan sulphate (Meyer and Chaffee, 1941; Pearce and Watson, 1949; Muir, 1964); they are present in similar amounts, although their ratio varies with age (Loewi and Meyer, 1958; Loewi, 1961). The absolute concentration of each in the dermis is very small: in man each represents 0·05% of the wet weight, in the pig 0·03%, and in the rat the combined amount is 0·09–0·12% (Smith, 1964). If ground substance makes up 50% of the skin's volume, the total polysaccharide concentration within it is therefore 0·12–0·24% in these species.

Similar mucopolysaccharides are found in other connective tissues. The properties of hyaluronic acid have been studied in extracts of synovial fluid, umbilical cord and vitreous humour, from which it can be obtained with little fear of degradation. Under these circumstances the molecular weight is very large; Blix and Snellman (1947) found values in the range 200 000–500 000, Laurent *et al.* (1960) 800 000–1 300 000 and Fessler (1960) 1 200 000–10 000 000. Such molecules are thixotropically viscous (Ogston and Stanier, 1953), i.e. they are very viscous until the fluid is in motion when they line up in the direction of flow and lose most of their viscous resistance. The viscosity of synovial fluid is not reduced by the action of trypsin (Ropes *et al.*, 1947), so that in this fluid the polysaccharides do not appear to be attached to protein.

The viscosity and molecular weight of the dermal polysaccharides are not known directly, because they are difficult to extract from the tissue and may therefore be degraded during extraction. However, hyaluronidase greatly increases the ease of diffusion through dermis (McLean and Hale, 1941) even allowing free movement of paramecia (Bensley, 1934). Hyaluronidase also increases the ease of fluid flow through the dermis (p. 81), although it does not increase the speed of viscous slip (p. 78).

In summary, the dermis is the load-bearing and compressible tissue in the skin. It contains a highly characterized fibrous protein which bears the load, and a less well-defined fluid which flows under pressure.

THEORY OF STRETCH AND COMPRESSION

EXTENSION

The extensibility of skin is a measure of the extensibility of the collagen within it (p. 81). Once the initial slack has been exhausted, it is a measure of the extensibility of the actual collagen fibrils. Most collagen fibrils in dermis lie parallel to the skin surface, but may lie in any direction within this plane. Thus pulling the skin in any one direction is likely to extend only a fraction of the fibrils. This fraction is unknown; I have assumed it to be one-half. On these assumptions, the elastic modulus for skin collagen (Y_c) may be calculated from the observed values for skin (Y):

$$Y_c = \frac{2Y}{\alpha} \tag{8a}$$

For a fully orientated system
$$Y_c = \frac{Y}{\alpha} \tag{8b}$$

Where α = volume fraction of the skin which is collagen.

Hence for rat skin $Y_c = 16 \times 10^8$ dynes/cm², for human skin $32\text{--}73 \times 10^8$ dynes/cm²; α is unknown for pig skin, but if $\alpha = 0.2$, then $Y_c = 26\text{--}29 \times 10^8$ dynes/cm². In tendon all the fibrils are orientated parallel to the axis of the tendon, so that equation 8b holds. If one assumes that in the juvenile tendons studied by Burton (1954) and Bull (1957) $\alpha = 0.5$, then in tendon $Y_c = 14\text{--}26 \times 10^8$ dynes/cm². Thus collagen in skin appears to be as strong as, or stronger than, juvenile tendon collagen; Burton noted that the tendons of older animals were stronger, so that no significance can be given to the difference. All the limited data show that collagen fibrils in skin can be extended by 10–30% of their length before they break, and that during this extension they are as strong as the same structures elsewhere. More detailed and precise data would be very interesting, since there is a clear variation of Y_c with age, and this parameter is presumably a measure of cross-linkage within the collagen fibril. It is particularly interesting that although the cross-linkage in skin collagen appears to rise with age, it can still be extended by approximately the same proportion of its resting length before rupture.

When skin is slack its extensibility is clearly not a property of the bulk of its collagen, the fibrils of which are presumably bent. The slack is not due to re-orientation of fibrils within the plane of the skin, for otherwise there would be no slack in the diaphragm preparation. The extensibility of slack skin may be as great as $100 \times$ that of tense skin (Fig. 32). Dick (1951) has suggested that the elastin is responsible for these small restoring forces, and that the collagen is irrelevant to the tonic tension in skin. There are two reasons for this hypothesis: firstly, collagen is known to slip under larger maintained forces (Harkness and Harkness, 1959a), and secondly the restoring force at low extension is correlated with the elastin content of the skin (Dick, 1951). However, elastin is extremely extensible (in the ligamentum nuchae $Y = 0.25 \times 10^8$ dynes/cm^2, Bull (1957); if $\alpha = 0.5$, applying equation 8b, $Y_e = 0.5 \times 10^8$ dynes/cm^2), and there is only 1% of elastin by volume in the skin. Thus elastin of the kind present in ligamentum nuchae could only provide a skin elastic modulus of 0.005×10^8 dynes/cm^2, which would not account for even the first part of the stress-strain curve. Either the skin elastin is stronger, or the collagen will withstand a small tension indefinitely.

Viscous slip under higher tension is a property of many collagenous tissues (Harkness and Harkness, 1959a). The extremely exact molecular orientation and spacing within the collagen fibril make slip within it an unlikely event. Either the individual fibrils slip relative to one another, or the whole sets, the histological fibres, do so. In either case, the system is similar to that in which an array of rods in a viscous medium is slowly pulled apart (Fig. 42). A particular case of such motion, in which all the rods are equally spaced, and overlap by half their length, is examined in detail in Appendix III. By making a rough approximation for the viscous force between the rods, one obtains the following relation for the viscous extensibility:

$$u = \frac{v}{l_0 T}$$

$$= \frac{4h^2 (h - 2r)}{\pi \eta x^2 r} \tag{9}$$

See Fig. 42 for meanings of symbols, and Appendix III for derivation of the equation.

The viscosity of the ground substance is unknown, and is probably critically dependent on the velocity gradient due to the motion within it, since this determines the orientation, and hence viscosity, of the macromolecules. In the case of the slow viscous slip the velocity gradient is probably less than the critical value necessary for this orientation, approx. 10 sec^{-1} (Ogston and Stanier, 1953). These authors found that at <1 sec^{-1} synovial hyaluronic acid gave $\eta = 2$–$1\,000$ cpoise in the concentration range $0\cdot1$–$0\cdot5\%$, which is probably near that in the ground substance. However, it is known that hyaluronic acid is not itself responsible for restraining the viscous slip (Harkness and Harkness, 1959a), and chondroitin sulphate is more closely connected to the dermal collagen than hyaluronic acid (Rothman, 1954). It is

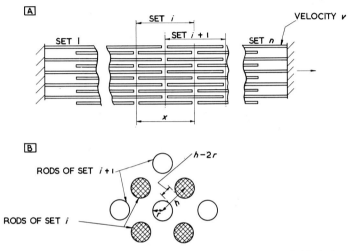

FIG. 42. A system of regularly spaced rods moving in a viscous fluid. A, longitudinal section; B, transverse section.

therefore impossible to predict the value of η in the ground substance, and both extreme assumptions, $\eta = 1$ cpoise and $\eta = 10^4$ cpoise, have been used to bracket the possible behaviour. The viscous extensibility of rat skin is 10^{-11} cm^2/dyne sec (p. 78). By applying likely values for the radius and inter-centre spacing of the fibrils and fibres to equation 9 one can see whether the model could provide the observed viscous resistance. Thus fibres of radius 5 μ, separated by 1 μ, would need to be 20 cm ($\eta = 10^4$ cpoise) or 2 000 cm ($\eta = 1$ cpoise) long to provide the resistance. This is ridiculous; one has to assume that the histological fibres form a continuous syncytium. Even interfibrillar dimensions require a high viscosity to account for the observed resistance: fibrils 500 Å in radius and spaced by 100 Å would need to be $0\cdot2$ cm ($\eta = 10^4$ cpoise) or 20 cm ($\eta = 1$ cpoise) long. Only the first of these is reasonable. On this model, therefore, one must assume that the slip is interfibrillar, that the interfibrillar ground substance is highly viscous and that the collagen fibrils are very long. The only other way of explaining the lack of slip in the collagen would be to assume a high degree of fibril coiling, for which the electron microscope gives no support; there are no "knots" which hold the fibrils together, therefore they must hold by fluid friction.

The sudden breakdown when the ultimate tensile stress is reached may be due to a reduction in viscosity of the macromolecules as soon as the fluid begins to move.

COMPRESSION

Compression of skin is primarily due to flow of ground substance through the dermis, between the collagen fibrils or fibres. The only mathematical treatment available of viscous flow in a compressed system is the flow of liquid out from between two parallel plates (Reynolds, 1886, quoted by Barr, 1931). Movement between plates is qualitatively similar to movement between fibres, because as the system is compressed, it is only the vertical dimension of the fibre mat which is reduced (and gradually comes to dominate the resistance). The plate system is therefore a plausible model for dermal compression. A particular case, a set of stacks of such plates, has been considered in Appendix IV and is illustrated in Fig. 43. This case was chosen because of the power relationship between area of application and speed of deformation found by Tregear and Dirnhuber (1965): they found that the speed of deformation for a given pressure fell only slightly with increase of area from $0.1-4.0 \text{ cm}^2$. Thus it appeared that the viscous resistance was in comparatively short channels; if the channels had extended right across the compressed area, increase of the area would have greatly increased the effective resistance and thus decreased the speed of deformation for a given pressure. During viscous flow in the dermis (Fig. 35, p. 80) there is an initial rapid flow while the channels are wide, and a long "tail" after they have become narrow. It is a completely different time-course from the common biological exponential. In mathematical terms:

$$\frac{h}{h_0} = \sqrt{\frac{1}{1+\beta t}} \tag{10}*$$

where
$$\beta = \frac{16 F x_0^2}{3 \pi^2 \eta a^2 r^2} \tag{11}$$

(see Fig. 43 for meaning of symbols, and Appendix IV for derivation).

The time taken to reach $h = \frac{h_0}{2}$, $t_{\frac{1}{2}}$, is given by:

$$t_{\frac{1}{2}} = \frac{9 \pi^2 \eta r^2 a^2}{16 F x_0^2} \tag{12}$$

* This equation was misprinted in the text of Tregear and Dirnhuber (1965); the square root sign was omitted.

Tregear and Dirnhuber found that a 1 kg weight ($F \fallingdotseq 10^6$ dynes) applied over a circle of radius 0·4 cm took approx. 2·5 min to reach a 50% deformation. If one assumes $\eta = 100$ cpoise, a mean value between the extremes used in the previous calculation, then channels 12 000 × as long as they were wide would be needed to account for the observed resistance to flow: 1 μ channels would have to be 12 mm long, 100 Å channels 120 μ long. If $\eta = 10^4$ cpoise, then the channels would only have to be 1 200 × as long as wide. Thus again,

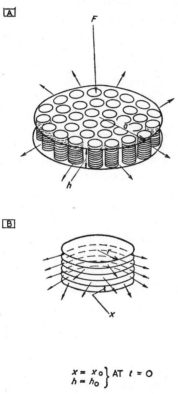

$$\begin{aligned} x &= x_0 \\ h &= h_0 \end{aligned} \right\} \text{AT } t = 0$$

Fig. 43. Set of stacks of circular plates containing a viscous liquid, compressed by a vertical force. B, Single stack.

the calculation indicates that the ground substance behaves as a very viscous material. In this instance, however, the hyaluronic acid appears to be the viscous macromolecule (Fig. 36). The calculation in itself does not allow a clear choice between the alternatives of interfibrillar or interfibre movement; in any case it is probably incorrect to apply the model to dimensions much less than 1 μ, because ultrafiltration is likely to occur (Fessler, 1960).

These three theoretical treatments, of elastic extension, viscous extension and viscous compression, are of necessity brief and simple. The data on which

F

they are based are few, and not very accurate. Nevertheless, the most obvious features of the structure of the dermis do appear to explain the most obvious features of the skin's mechanical function.

MECHANICAL PROPERTIES OF THE EPIDERMIS

The epidermis is a comparatively strong structure, for despite the fact that it is only 0·1 mm thick, it holds together when under pressure from blister fluid. Its strength is probably due to its intercellular bridge and intracellular fibril system (p. 32). Under most general tension on the skin the epidermis itself is unstretched, because at rest it is covered by an elaborate system of organized folds (Horstmann and Dabelow, 1957).

The dermo-epidermal junction is a weak point in skin, particularly human skin. It can be broken apart by direct negative pressure (Kiistalla and Mustakallio, 1964) or by a variety of chemical and physical injuries (Baumberger et al., 1941). The junction consists of a "basement membrane", an osmiophil band 200–400 Å thick (Pearson and Spargo, 1962) crossed by fine fibrils in desmosome-like structures (Breathnack, 1964). The region has a high polysaccharide content (Dodson, 1963). Felsher (1947) showed that many blistering agents act on the superficial collagen of the dermis, which appears to be particularly easy to weaken; it is certainly formed of much smaller groups of fibrils, or histological fibres (Jacobson, 1953). When the basement membrance itself separates from the epidermal cells it moves as one piece (Pearson and Spargo, 1962), indicating adhesion along its entire surface and not just at the desmosome-like areas.

PRACTICAL IMPLICATIONS

Each of the general mechanical properties of the skin have obvious practical implications. The slack in skin allows it to stretch around moving joints without slowing their movement. The high strength of skin once the slack is taken up prevents its breakage except under extreme stress. In the largest mammals, notable the pachyderms, the dermis is particularly thick over the torso, where the force exerted by the weight of the abdominal contents must be considerable. In the small, densely furred rodents, where there is very little stress from the animal's own weight, and the hair distributes external stresses, the skin is extremely thin (Fig. 37). The effects of the breakdown of skin strength are seen in cutis laxa and in senile elastosis.

Viscous slip under tension certainly occurs in rapid growths, such as boils, and may be the normal means of allowing for body growth. Its irreversibility is strikingly shown in starvation; the skin does not shrink to fit the body beneath it. Striae gravidae are presumably a case in which the slip has been so rapid that the fibril overlap has broken down, and hence the viscous force limiting further slip has been lost.

Viscous flow in skin is seen whenever a small object is gripped or pressed (e.g. a rope) or when a subject is immobile for a long time, when his own weight causes the flow. It has the effect of moulding the skin around the object which is exerting the force, and thus reducing the pressure on any one point.

CHAPTER 4

Photons and Molecules
The Absorption of Radiation by Skin

Electromagnetic radiation consists of photons which are both waves and particles. As a wave, a photon is characterized by its wavelength; as a particle, it is characterized by its quantum of energy. The energy of the photon is inversely proportional to its wavelength ($E = 12\,400/\lambda$ where E is in electron-volts (eV) and λ is in Angstrom units (Å)). It is usual to think of high-energy photons such as X-rays in terms of their quantum energy, because they behave more as particles and less as waves, while the comparatively low-energy photons of ultraviolet, visible and infrared radiation behave as waves, and are specified by their wavelength.

Any oscillating charged particle will create photons; a selection of sources is shown in Table XVII. The two classes of photon which are important relative to skin are the high-energy particles (X, γ and cosmic rays) and the low-energy particles (ultraviolet, visible and infrared radiation). Between these two disparate wavebands there is a large gap of wavelengths which are not present in nature, and are not readily produced.

The low-energy waveband may usefully be subdivided in terms of its effect on the skin, rather than its visibility. Only radiation of wavelength less than 3 150 Å, i.e. particle energy in excess of 4 eV, will produce the erythema of sunburn (Coblentz *et al.*, 1932). Such radiation is often termed "erythematous", and the rest is "non-erythematous".

In the treatment which follows, the absorption by skin of, first, low-energy and, second, high-energy radiation is described, followed by a brief description of the after-effects of absorption.

THE TRANSFER OF LOW-ENERGY RADIATION THROUGH SKIN

PRINCIPLES

When radiation reaches a surface it is reflected or transmitted. On further passage through the bulk of the material the radiation may be absorbed or scattered (deviated); scattering is strong in inhomogeneous materials. Skin is inhomogeneous, and a great deal of the light transmitted through it is scattered in transit (Hardy *et al.*, 1956). Scattering has two separable effects: firstly, the average path traversed by the light is greater than the thickness of the

TABLE XVII. *Some natural and artificial radiation sources*

Source	Waveband or quantal energy
Bulk electron vibrator	
Radio	10–1 000 m
Radar	0·1–10 cm
Thermal molecular energy	
Sun	0·3–3 μ
Surroundings	3–30 μ*
Electrically excited molecular energy	
Mercury discharge tube	2 537, 2 967, 3 020, 3 130 Å
Crystal lattice vibration	
Ruby laser	6 943 Å
Electronic impact	
X-ray tube	0·01–5 Å (2 keV–1 MeV)
Nuclear rearrangement	
γ-emitting isotope	0·001–0·1 Å (0·1–10 MeV)
Solar electron impact	
Cosmic rays	5×10^{-7}–5×10^{-6} Å (2 000–20 000 MeV)

* This is an exchange between skin and its environment. N.B. 10 000 Å = 1 μ; 10 000 μ = 1 cm.

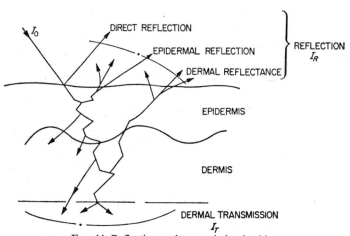

FIG. 44. Reflection and transmission in skin.

layer of tissue itself, and secondly, some of the light is turned through more than 90° and re-emerges from the skin as reflected light (Fig. 44). Thus skin reflection is a function in depth, not a surface phenomenon. This makes measurements of reflection (and absorption) more difficult to interpret than is the case for the homogeneous materials usual in physical optics, in which reflection occurs at the surface and only absorption occurs in the material itself. Nevertheless, the basic measurements remain the same. Reflection is defined by the reflectance (R):

$$R = I_R/I_0 \tag{1}$$

$$\text{where} \quad I_0 = \text{intensity of incident radiation}$$
$$I_R = \text{intensity of reflected radiation.}$$

Transmission is similarly defined by the transmittance

$$T = I_T/I_0 \tag{2}$$

$$\text{where} \quad I_T = \text{intensity of transmitted radiation.}$$

Since much of both the reflected and transmitted light is scattered, it is necessary to collect the light emerging in all directions in order to obtain I_R and I_T.

In homogeneous materials it is usual to calculate the absorption coefficient (μ) or its reciprocal the "space constant" (λ) from the transmittance, according to the equation

$$I_T = I_0 e^{-\mu x} \tag{3a}$$
$$= I_0 e^{-x/\lambda} \tag{3b}$$

For inhomogeneous materials such as skin the absorption coefficient is expected to be higher than it would be in homogeneous material containing the same absorbent compounds, for the light path is greater. The parameter is therefore little used. Nevertheless, the relation between transmittance and wavelength can be used to deduce the source of the absorption.

Since skin reflection occurs principally within the body of the skin, reflectance also is affected by absorption, and its relation to wavelength is used to detect absorption by skin components; indeed this is the more sensitive measurement of the two and can be performed *in vivo*. However, it is impossible to relate reflectance to absorption by skin components quantitatively, because the depth of penetration before reflection is indeterminate (unlike the depth in transmission measurements).

Techniques

The main difficulty in measuring absorption or reflection from the skin is in collecting all, or a representative sample, of the diffusely scattered radiation emitted from the under- or upper-surface of the tissue.

The methods used to measure skin absorption and reflection have varied enormously in complexity and sensitivity (for the two extremes, compare Martin, 1930; Clark *et al.*, 1953) but they can basically be classified according to how they attempt to overcome this difficulty.

Methods in which all the Light is Collected

The simplest way of collecting and measuring all the light transmitted through skin is to place the skin on a photographic plate (Fig. 45A). This automatically collects and integrates light coming from all directions. The method was used by many of the earlier workers (e.g. Lucas, 1930; Bachem

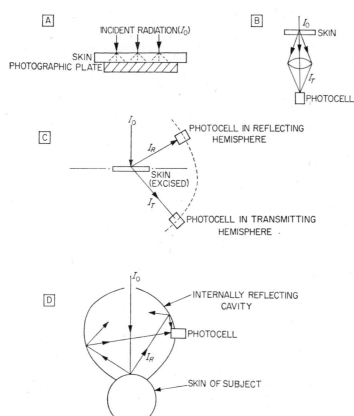

FIG. 45. Methods of measuring skin transmission and reflection.

and Reed, 1931). Its use is limited by the sensitivity of the photographic plate, and obviously it cannot be used to measure reflection.

A much more complex, and accurate, method which also effectively collects all the transmitted or reflected light is the goniometric spectrophotometer of Clark et al. (1953). In this instrument a monochromatic beam of light impinges on a piece of excised skin around which a photocell is moved on spherical co-ordinates (Fig. 45C). The integrated reading of the photocell for all positions in the hemisphere behind the specimen gives the total transmission, and integration over the other hemisphere gives the reflection. The individual readings show the type and degree of scattering produced in reflection and transmission. Since many readings must be taken at each wavelength, measurements on this instrument are bound to be lengthy. It is, however, an "absolute" instrument; it does not require preliminary standardization.

Methods in which the Light is Sampled

The most usual way of sampling is by accepting only a limited angle of the transmitted or reflected light (e.g. Kirby-Smith *et al.*, 1942a; Goldzieher *et al.*, 1951; Fig. 45B). Such measurements can be related to the total transmitted or reflected intensity only if the law relating angle of emission to intensity is known, or can be assumed. For reflection, and for transmission through full-thickness skin, Hardy *et al.* (1956) have shown that Lambert's cosine law ($I = k \cos \theta$, where θ = angle between the normal to the skin surface and the direction of emission) is obeyed. For such measurements sampling methods are therefore appropriate. For transmission through thin specimens such as epidermis, Lambert's law does not apply, and sampling becomes very difficult to apply accurately.

There is one device in which light reflected from all angles is sampled and automatically integrated. This is the integrating sphere. It consists of a cavity, not necessarily spherical, coated internally with a good diffuse reflector. A monochromatic beam of light enters the cavity and is reflected off the skin, which is apposed to another hole in the cavity wall (Fig. 45D). Some of the reflected light finally impinges on a photocell which is also mounted in the wall. This is not an "absolute" device, since the reflectance is deduced by comparing the reflection from skin to that from known reflectors, and these, in turn, have proved difficult to calibrate exactly (Hardy *et al.*, 1956). Also, it must be assumed that the skin reflection obeys Lambert's law. Nevertheless, an instrument designed by Jacquez and Kuppenheim (1955) has been used by their group to make very reproducible and spectrally precise measurements of skin reflectance. Its advantages are its speed of operation, spectral precision and ease of use with live subjects. Jacquez *et al.* (1955d) have examined the theory of the integrating sphere in detail.

TRANSMISSION THROUGH FUR AND THE LAYERS OF SKIN

Fur

It is generally assumed that dense fur transmits no radiation, although there have been no direct experiments to prove this. The reasons behind the assumption are that a thin layer of fur will transmit no visible light, and it is known that a water-protein mixture transmits radiation most easily in the visible waveband. MacFarlane *et al.* (1956) noted that under intense solar irradiation the outside of a sheep's fleece rose in temperature to near the boiling-point of water while the inside remained cool, which indicated that little penetration occurred. The lower limit of hair density below which radiation transfer through fur becomes appreciable is presumably that below which the skin is visible through the fur; this is in the range 100–1 000 hairs/cm^2 (Tregear, 1965a). The optical properties of skin itself are therefore only important in lightly haired or unhaired regions of mammals.

EPIDERMIS

Measurements of transmission have been made on keratinized epidermal membranes (Pearson and Gair, 1931; Mitchell, 1938; Scheuplein, 1964), on epidermis itself (Lucas, 1930; Hardy and Muschenheim, 1934; Kirby-Smith *et al.*, 1942a) and on epidermis with some dermis attached (Hardy *et al.*, 1956). The detailed results are not all mutually consistent, but the broad outlines of epidermal absorption are agreed. Untanned human epidermis transmits most of the incident light in the waveband 4 000–10 000 Å (the visible and very near infrared), little in the ultraviolet, and a variable amount in the further infrared (Fig. 46). Epidermal scattering is incomplete, i.e. much of the incident radiation is transmitted with little deviation in direction, as through a lightly ground glass plate (Hardy *et al.*, 1956).

The very high transmission of visible radiation by untanned human epidermis is greatly reduced by suntan (Fig. 47), and the transmission through heavily pigmented Negro epidermis is much less; Thomson (1955) showed that the membranes formed from cantharides blisters of African epidermis transmitted less than half as much as Europeans, although they were no thicker.

The epidermal transmission of 1–3 μ infrared light is appreciable, but is reduced by strong absorption bands (Fig. 46). These can be assigned to water absorption (p. 106). Above 3 μ, absorption is nearly complete (Hardy and Muschenheim, 1934; Scheuplein, 1964).

In the near ultraviolet waveband epidermal transmission falls rapidly as the wavelength is reduced (Fig. 47). Below 3 000 Å human epidermis transmits very little radiation, while mouse ear epidermis transmits approx. 4% down to 2 500 Å (Kirby-Smith *et al.*, 1942a), where there is a small peak in transmission. Below 2 500 Å epidermis transmits virtually no radiation (Bachem and Reed, 1931). If scattering is abolished by clearing the tissue in acetic acid or glycerol, ultraviolet transmission through human epidermis is greatly increased (Lucas, 1930) but the strong absorption band at 2 800 Å remains (Fig. 47).

One can increase the epidermal absorption of ultraviolet radiation by

F*

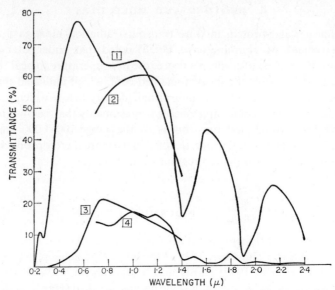

FIG. 46. Transmission of radiation through the epidermis (1; Bachem and Reed, 1931), a 400 μ thick layer including the epidermis (2; Hardy *et al.*, 1956), and a 1·6–2 mm thick layer of dermis (3, 4; Hardy *et al.*, 1956).

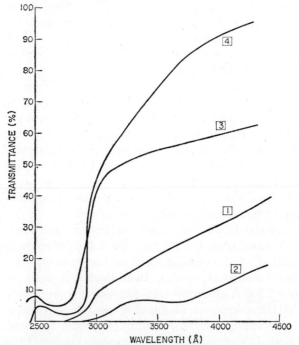

FIG. 47. Transmission of erythematous radiation through epidermis. (1) Untanned human epidermis; (2) tanned human epidermis; (3) mouse ear epidermis; (4) human epidermis cleared in acetic acid. (1–3, from Kirby-Smith *et al.*, 1942a; 4, from Lucas, 1930.)

inducing suntan (Fig. 47) or by adding aromatic compounds to the top surface; Stevanovic (1960) showed that a 50 μ-thick film of 5% p-aminobenzoic acid removed 99% of 2 900–3 200 Å radiation, and other benzene ring compounds have a similar effect. It was postulated that sweat may form an ultraviolet filter due to its aromatic content, but Crew and Whittle (1938) showed that in physiologically occurring thickness sweat was ineffective in absorbing ultraviolet radiation.

The thick epidermis of the palms and soles probably absorbs most infrared radiation, due to its high protein content. Some visible radiation is certainly transmitted, as the colour of the blood can be seen reflected from deeper layers.

DERMIS

The dermis absorbs or reflects nearly all the radiation transmitted through the epidermis. A small fraction of the red and near infrared radiation is transmitted through 2 mm of skin (Fig. 46) and presumably reaches the subcutaneous tissue *in vivo*. This fraction is probably much larger in exceptionally thin-skinned animals, such as hairless mice (Dimitroff *et al.*, 1955). The radiation transmitted through thick dermis is perfectly scattered (Hardy *et al.*, 1956). The absorption coefficient, or absorption per unit thickness, of dermis is less than that of the surface layers of skin for visible light, but is the same for infrared radiation (Hardy *et al.*, 1956).

REFLECTION FROM FUR AND SKIN

FUR

Fur absorbs perfectly in the far infrared, whatever its colour (Hammel, 1956); it therefore reflects no radiation in the waveband 4–40 μ. In the visible and near infrared, fur reflects considerably. Riemerschmid and Elder (1945) showed that the net reflectance of solar radiation from white cow hair was 50%, and Stewart *et al.* (1951) showed that the spectral reflectance of albino rat hair rose to a maximum of 80% at 7 000 Å; the reflectance was much less at shorter wavelengths (Fig. 49). Coloured fur reflects much less radiation than white fur: black cows reflected only 8% of the incident solar radiation (Riemerschmid and Elder, 1945). These figures refer to light falling vertically on the fur, as do all the subsequent figures for skin. If the radiation was presented to the fur at a grazing incidence reflection was much greater. The thickness or orientation of the pelt had no appreciable effect on its reflectance.

SKIN

Like fur, skin reflects a great deal of visible and near infrared radiation, and very little ultraviolet or far infrared radiation (Hardy and Muschenheim, 1934). The net reflectance of solar radiation from a blond human skin is in the region of 30–40% (Martin, 1930; Oppel and Hardy, 1937). It is highly dependent on the skin colour; a dark Negro skin reflected only 16%. Reflection of visible light is a phenomenon in depth; 0·4 mm thick excised skin reflected only half that reflected by a 2 mm thick specimen (Hardy et al., 1956). On the other hand, the slight reflection (5–10%) usually found in the ultraviolet and far infrared is probably a surface reflection (Dimitroff et al., 1955) since any radiation of these wavebands which penetrated into the skin would be likely to be absorbed before it could be reflected.

The spectral reflectance of white human skin has been determined by several observers (Fig. 48). The results are not in complete agreement; Hardy et al. (1956) found a significantly lower reflection of infrared radiation from excised skin than did Jacquez et al. (1955 b, c) from intact skin, and Edwards et al. (1951) obtained curiously low reflectance values in the visible region. Nevertheless, the main features of reflection by white human skin have been established. The maximum reflectance is 60–70%, at 7 000 Å, the boundary between the visible and the infrared. As the wavelength is increased, reflection declines, with marked dips at the same absorption bands seen in transmission measurements (Figs. 46 and 48). Above 2 μ the only reflection is a small, presumably surface, reflection. Below 7 000 Å the reflectance declines as the wavelength is reduced, and this curve is also indented by sharp and highly characteristic dips (Fig. 48). These can be assigned to absorption bands of haemoglobin and, less certainly, of carotene (Edwards et al., 1951). Three independent observations of reflectance by white human skin in the visible and ultraviolet show remarkably good mutual agreement (Fig. 48).

Reflection of visible and ultraviolet light by the unpigmented skin of other species is similar to that of white human skin (Fig. 49, lines, 2, 4 and 5). The characteristic absorption bands of haemoglobin are clearly visible, and on cyanosis their maxima change to the wavelengths of reduced haemoglobin (Jacquez et al., 1955a). Negro skin reflects much less visible or ultraviolet light (Fig. 49), and suntanning of white subjects also reduces the reflectance of visible light (Kuppenheim and Heer, 1952). In the near infrared, however, both suntanned (Kuppenheim and Heer, 1952) and Negro (Hardy et al., 1956) skin reflect the same amount as untanned white skin.

THEORY OF ABSORPTION AND REFLECTION BY SKIN

The sharp epidermal absorption of radiation of wavelengths less than 3 200 Å (Fig. 47), and the accompanying reduction in skin reflection (Fig. 49), are both signs of an absorption band. It has been conclusively shown that

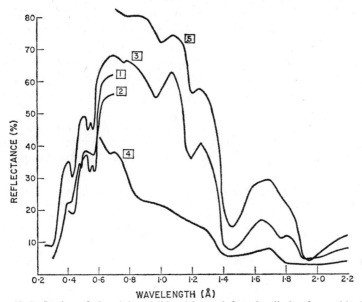

FIG. 48. Reflection of ultraviolet, visible and near infrared radiation from white human skin. Data of (1) Edwards and Duntley (1939); (2) Goldzieher *et al.* (1951); (3) Jacquez *et al.* (1955 b, c); (4) Hardy *et al.* (1956). The reflection from a 35% MgO paste in water (Jacquez *et al.*, 1955c) is also shown (5).

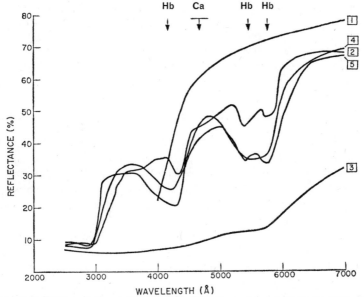

FIG. 49. Reflection of ultraviolet and visible light from white rabbit fur (1; Stewart *et al.*, 1951), white (2) and Negro (3) human skin (Jacquez *et al.*, 1955c), pig skin (4; Kuppenheim *et al.*, 1956), and white rabbit skin (5; Dimitroff *et al.*, 1955). The absorption maxima of haemoglobin (Hb) and carotene (Ca) are marked above.

this absorption is due to the aromatic amino acids of the epidermal protein. Thus Lucas (1930) showed that tryptophan or tyrosine solution produced a 2 800 Å-maximum absorption band which mimicked the transmission of cleared stratum corneum, and Mitchell (1938) showed that the absorption was quantitatively equivalent to 50 μ thickness of a 6% protein solution. Similarly Blum and Terus (1946) equated epidermal absorption to that of a 10 μ-thick 10% phenyl salicylate solution.

Relatively few of the amino acids in keratin are aromatic (Matoltsy, 1958) but the protein is so concentrated in the stratum corneum that the net aromatic content is high. The complete absorption of ultraviolet radiation of

TABLE XVIII. *Absorption maxima of some compounds present in skin*

Compound	Wavelength	Author
Tyrosine ⎫ Tryptophan ⎭	2 800 Å	Lucas (1930)
Carotene	4 550–4 850 Å	⎫
Haemoglobin	3 500 Å	
	4 170 Å	
	5 480 Å	
	5 780 Å	Edwards *et al.* (1951)
Reduced haemoglobin	4 310 Å	
	5 650 Å	
Melanin	3 000–6 000 + Å	⎭
Water	0·76 μ (7 600 Å)	Jacquez *et al.* (1955 a, b)
	0·84 μ	
	0·96 μ	
	1·2 μ	
	1·45 μ	
	1·9 μ	
	2·4 μ	

less than 2 500 Å is largely due to absorption by the peptide linkages themselves (Haurowitz, 1963).

The absorption bands seen *by reflectance* in the visible and near ultraviolet can be assigned to haemoglobin and carotene. Haemoglobin has sharp absorption peaks (Table XVIII) at least three of which are clearly visible by reflection (Fig. 49), and shift appropriately on reduction of the pigment. A fourth, the 3 500 Å band, has been tentatively ascribed to a reflectance dip (Jacquez and Kuppenheim, 1954). Carotene has a broader absorption band (Table XVIII) to which a flattening of the reflectance curve of human skin can be ascribed (Fig. 49). Edwards *et al.* (1951) satisfied themselves that this flattening disappeared on extraction of carotene. The flattening is absent in reflection from animal skin (Jacquez *et al.*, 1955a). Melanin absorbs over the whole visible and near ultraviolet waveband, without sharp peaks (Edwards *et al.*, 1951); this is due to its complex condensed ring structure (Daniels, 1959). In Negro skin its strong absorption in the epidermis prevents adequate transmission to the dermis for the haemoglobin reflectance peaks to appear (Fig. 49).

The series of absorption bands in the near infrared seen both in transmission (Fig. 46) and reflection (Fig. 48) can all be assigned to the absorption of water (Table XVIII). Jacquez *et al.* (1955c) produced a reasonably good quantitative simulation of skin reflection in the near infrared from a reflecting paste in water (Fig. 48). Since absorption of near infrared radiation is mainly due to water, it may be assumed to take place uniformly throughout all hydrated structures, irrespective of their histological content. This agrees with the observation that the absorption coefficient of dermis is the same as that of epidermis in the near infrared, although they differ in the visible waveband (Hardy *et al.*, 1956).

In the far infrared absorption is again mainly due to protein. Hardy and Muschenheim (1934) showed that epidermal absorption in the far infrared was similar to that of triethylamine, and Scheuplein has analysed the intramolecular components of the protein which are responsible for absorption. He finds that methylene and amide linkages are particularly strong absorbents of the far infrared radiation.

SUMMARY

The skin absorbs nearly all far ultraviolet radiation, reflecting a little from its surface. In the 2 800 Å region this absorption is due to benzene rings. Above 3 000 Å an appreciable fraction of the incoming radiation penetrates deeply enough to be scattered and partially reflected in depth. Hence the reflectance rises as the penetration deepens. Where skin compounds absorb a specific wavelength the reflection is reduced, and presumably penetration is also weakened. Penetration and reflection are maximum in the red end of the visible spectrum, where the radiation penetrates 1–3 mm, and most of it is eventually reflected out again. This is a true reflection in depth. In heavily pigmented skin most radiation is absorbed near the surface so that neither penetration nor its concomitant reflection can occur.

In the near infrared the skin water absorbs strongly, limiting penetration and reflection, and in the far infrared resonances within the proteins cause almost perfect absorption within the surface layers of the skin.

ABSORPTION OF HIGH-ENERGY RADIATION BY SKIN

High-energy radiation interacts with matter by ionization, and its intensity is cited in terms of the energy absorbed by ionization. The unit employed is the rad, which is the radiation needed to produce 100 ergs energy absorbed per gram of tissue. This measure of absorbed energy can be used to calculate the incident energy flux (Appendix V) but the calculation is of little use, since the effect of the radiation is directly dependent on the ionization, and not on the incident energy.

Transmission of high-energy radiation is measured by the ionization produced in a detector behind the tissue. A large variety of such detectors have been developed (Faires and Parkes, 1960). Reflection and scattering are relatively slight so that the transmission measurements are simpler to interpret than is the case for low-energy radiation.

The ease of transmission of a given radiation is described by the space constant (λ; equation 3b, p. 98) which is the thickness of tissue required to reduce the intensity to 37% (1/e) of its original value.

Interaction between high-energy radiation and matter takes place deep within the electron shell of the atoms (Grodstein, 1957), so that it is only dependent on the atomic weights of the atoms present in the tissue and not on their chemical configuration. There is therefore only slight variation in the absorption of a given radiation by different tissues, except for those containing many heavy atoms, like bone (Spiers, 1946); for all high-energy radiation skin may be considered as a homogeneous absorber.

The space constants of absorption of high-energy radiation in excess of 50 keV are all considerably greater than the thickness of normal mammalian skin (Grodstein, 1957; Cohen, 1961). Irradiation of skin by such particles is therefore virtually uniform.

Particles of lower energy are much more readily absorbed in tissue, so that their space constant is less than the thickness of the skin. Irradiation of skin by such particles is not uniform (Cohen, 1961). The Grenz X-rays used in skin therapy are mostly absorbed within 0·5 mm of the skin surface (Fig. 50; Vennart, 1954), so that subcutaneous tissue receives little radiation. Even the softest X-rays penetrate the epidermis, so that there is no dermis-sparing X-radiation available.

In addition to photons, radioisotopes produce two types of charged particle. Of these, the α-particles are so rapidly absorbed by tissue that they do not even reach the live epidermis (Newbery, 1964), while the β-particles irradiate either the epidermis only, or the skin as a whole, depending on their energy.

EFFECTS OF RADIATION ON SKIN

Radiation may affect skin by heating it up (bulk energy transfer) or by quantal transfer to individual molecules, provided the radiation quanta are large enough to disrupt the molecules.

HEAT BURNS

The only sources of energy which are capable of burning skin by heating it are hot bodies and pulsed light sources. The most formidable continuous sources of radiation are the sun and large fires, and the major sources of energy pulses are atomic bombs and lasers. At sea-level on earth the sun is equivalent to a black body at 6 000° K with nearly all the ultraviolet and

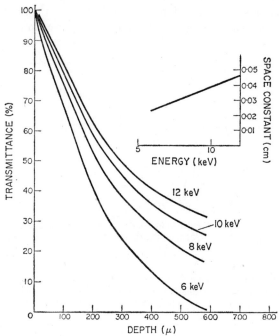

FIG. 50. Transmission of Grenz X-rays through skin. (Redrawn from Vennart, 1954.)

some of the infrared radiation removed (Fig. 51); its total irradiation does not exceed 1·4 cal/cm² min (Gates, 1962). Fires are usually at a lower temperature, but may subtend a much larger angle at the skin's surface and so irradiate it more intensely than the sun. Atomic bombs are briefly at a very high temperature, and may subtend a sufficient angle at the skin to produce a damaging pulse of thermal radiation, while the beam of a laser is so well collimated that all of its energy may be incident on a very small skin area, and so damage the skin.

Since heat is rapidly conducted, convected and radiated away from skin (see Chapter 5), a steady intensity of incident radiation soon reaches balance with heat loss, at an elevated skin surface temperature. Estimates of equilibration time vary between 1 and 10 min (Henriques and Moritz, 1947a;

Lipkin and Hardy, 1954). Epidermal damage occurs if the skin temperature is raised to 47° C for many minutes (Henriques and Moritz, 1947b); this normally requires an incident energy intensity of 6 cal/cm² min (Buettner, 1951). Since solar irradiation does not exceed 1·4 cal/cm² min sunlight itself will not, in normal circumstances, actually burn skin. Large fires, in forest or man-made holocausts, will do so. Since pain usually occurs before skin damage (Henriques and Moritz, 1947b), such steady irradiation is unlikely to cause damage unless it is impossible to get away from it.

A pulse of infrared radiation exceeding 2 cal/cm² will raise the skin temperature sufficiently to damage the epidermis (Morton *et al.*, 1952). The

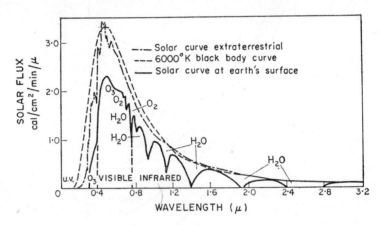

FIG. 51. Extra-terrestrial solar flux, the solar flux at the earth's surface, and the flux from a 6 000°K black body as a function of wavelength. The absorption bands resulting from atmospheric O_2, O_3 and H_2O are shown. (From Gates, 1962.)

energy must be delivered within 3 sec to have its full effect; longer exposures require more total energy to produce a burn, although lower rates of irradiation (Evans *et al.*, 1955). Visible light is only 60% as effective as infrared light in producing burns, presumably due to its greater reflection from the skin (Butterfield *et al.*, 1956). The area of irradiation is not critical for epidermal damage, but irradiation of wider areas produces more dermal damage (Morton *et al.*, 1952). Small laser beams producing pulses of 1–10 cal/cm² will also burn skin (Goldman *et al.*, 1963, 1964; Fine *et al.*, 1963).

A skin surface temperature in excess of 50° C is required to burn skin if the heating is only applied for a few seconds (Henriques and Moritz, 1947b). This means that 2 cal/cm² raise the skin surface by 20° C, i.e. the heat is distributed within approximately 1 mm of the tissue. A complete theory of heat transfer during and after radiation pulses has been developed and tested by Buettner (1951) and Hendler *et al.* (1958).

SUNBURN

Radiation of wavelengths less than 3 200 Å has a further effect on the skin than heating; its quantal energy (3·9 eV) is sufficient to disrupt the molecules individually. The first sign of this "sunburn" is a general reduction in enzyme activity within epidermal cells (Baden and Pearlman, 1964) followed, after

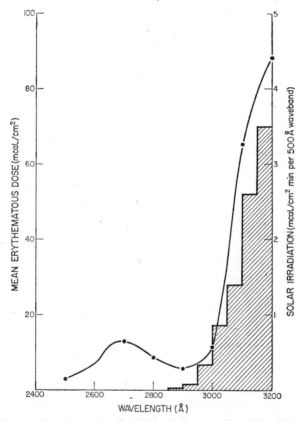

FIG. 52. The maximum intensity of sunlight in the near ultraviolet (shaded area; data from Petit, 1932) and the quantity required to produce sunburn erythema (Magnus, 1964).

some 4 h, by vasodilation in the dermis, "erythema" (Daniels *et al.*, 1961). In normal white human skin 2–30 mcal/cm² of 3 000 Å radiation are needed to produce erythema (Coblentz *et al.*, 1932; Blum *et al.*, 1946; Magnus, 1964). The radiation may be applied all at once, or spread over several minutes without loss of effect. Ultraviolet radiation of 2 500 or 3 000 Å is particularly erythematous; intermediate wavelengths are slightly less effective, and longer wavelengths are much less effective (Fig. 52).

Since very little, if any, 2 500–3 000 Å radiation reaches the dermis and enzyme changes are seen in irradiated epidermal cells, it is generally assumed that sunburn is an epidermal reaction, or reactions; there is no certainty that 2 500 Å and 3 000 Å radiation act in the same manner. The physiologically important process is the sunburn produced by the higher wavelength radiation, since no radiation less than 2 850 Å is present in sunlight (Fig. 52). It is not clear how much of the erythematous action of sunlight is due to the minute quantities of highly effective 2 850–3 050 radiation, and how much to the relatively gross but ineffective 3 050–3 300 Å radiation. Radiation of still longer wavelength is certainly totally ineffective, as otherwise full solar radiation would damage white skin in much less than the 20 min which is often quoted (Lorincz, 1960).

The primary epidermal reaction of sunburn is the formation of free radicals, and not ions, for the quantal energy available (3·9–4·2 eV) is similar to the energy of C-C and C-N bonds but is less than the ionization potential of water and peptides (Coulson, 1952). The reactant is probably protein, since the action spectrum of erythematous radiation parallels protein absorption, and not that of nucleic acid (Mitchell, 1938). The primary reaction is independent of temperature (Clark, 1936) or oxygen tension (Blum et al., 1935), unlike the response to high-energy particles. Melanin may reduce the reaction by acting as a radical trap, as well as a radiation absorber (Daniels, 1959). The substance which diffuses into the dermis after the primary reaction is not histamine (Partington, 1954); it appears to be a substance released from cells killed by the radiation (Soffen and Blum, 1961).

Much greater quantities of ultraviolet radiation also produce skin tumours; in white mice fibrosarcomas were produced by irradiating the skin with 50–100 cal/cm^2 of ultraviolet radiation (Kirby-Smith et al., 1942b). This reaction is cumulative over several months.

Light of wavelengths greater than 3 200 Å will damage hypersensitive human skin ("urticaria solaris"; Magnus and Porter, 1959; Blum et al., 1946; Ive et al., 1965), or normal skin to which a fluorescent substance (Blum et al., 1935) or psoralen (Pathak, 1962; Buck et al., 1960) has been added. A large amount of visible radiation will also cause hyperaemia in deep dermal blood vessels (Rottier and van der Leun, 1960). Prolonged exposure to mild sunlight eventually causes elastotic degeneration of the dermal collagen (Chapter 3, p. 87).

RADIATION BURNS AND SKIN TUMOURS

X-ray doses of greater than 200 rads usually cause direct skin damage. The first sign of the damage is an erythema, as in sunburn (Jelliffe, 1964; Zackheim et al., 1964). The erythema may be maintained for several days, and epidermal changes follow, often causing desquamation (Jelliffe, 1964) or alteration of the surface pattern (Harvey, 1954). In hairy mammals the dominant feature of the reaction to this mild irradiation is greying of the hair and epilation (Strauss *et al.*, 1954).

Larger, or repeated, doses of X-rays cause the development of skin carcinomas and sarcomas (Hulse, 1964). Grenz rays are less carcinogenic than the more energetic particles, presumably due to their limited range (Zackheim *et al.*, 1964).

The primary reaction of high-energy particles with tissue is an ionization (Grodstein, 1957). The further reactions which ensue are believed to be between free radicals (Howard-Flanders, 1958). Unlike the reactions in sunburn, radiation damage can be reduced or averted if the oxygen tension of the skin is reduced (Strauss *et al.*, 1954), or if the skin is cooled (Evans *et al.*, 1942). Certain compounds, notably cysteamine, will act as radiation protectors (Brinkman and Lambert, 1958).

The total energy of X-rays required to produce radiation damage is not much different from the ultraviolet energy necessary to produce sunburn (500 rads at 100 keV $\equiv$ 9 mcal/cm^2 (Appendix V); erythemal threshold for sunburn at 3 000 Å $\fallingdotseq$ 6 mcal/cm^2). However, little of the *incident* energy of the X-rays is absorbed in the skin, while practically all that of the ultraviolet radiation is absorbed in the epidermis; the space constant of 100 keV radiation is 6 cm, whilst that of 3 000 Å radiation is only some 0·003 cm. Thus the absolute effectiveness of the high-energy particles, in terms of damage produced per unit energy absorbed, is very much greater than that of ultraviolet radiation.

CHAPTER 5

Transfer of Molecular Kinetic Energy
Heat Loss through Skin

The flow of heat is the only physiologically regulated transfer through skin. Many, although not all, mammals keep their body temperature constant under widely varying climatic conditions, by varying their heat production and their thermal insulation. In the cold insulation is maximized by postural reduction in the exposed surface area, pilo-erection, reduction in cutaneous blood flow and countercurrent heat exchange between the arteries and veins. In the heat insulation is minimized by increase of exposed surface area and blood flow, and by evaporation from the skin surface and the mouth.

Heat flow is the transfer of random kinetic energy from one molecule to another. It is dependent on the degree of contact between molecules and does not require net transfer of the molecules themselves. Because of this thin layers of a material cannot act as near-perfect barriers to heat flow, as they can to diffusion. Thermal insulation is necessarily a relatively crude physical function, dependent on much thicker layers of tissue than have been considered in the previous chapters. Gases are much better insulators than liquids, and the still air within and above the fur is usually the most effective insulative layer. The main insulative layers beneath the skin surface are the fat, the connective tissue, and in limbs the whole structure along its length. The epidermis is too thin to be relevant.

In the following sections the transfer of heat by conduction and radiation through these various layers is first discussed, and the mechanism of evaporative heat loss from the skin surface is described separately. Finally the various parts of the system are reassembled to demonstrate their relative importance in animals under cold stress and heat stress.

CONDUCTION AND CONVECTION

PRINCIPLES

Thermal conduction is the transfer of energy by the interaction of molecules singly, thermal convection the transfer when molecules move in groups carrying their energy with them. In air both processes occur. In free air a slight wind makes convection dominant, and even in the absence of wind a warm surface causes convection. Within fur, convection is greatly obstructed. In tissue, the molecules are not so readily convected, and heat flow is by conduction, plus the controlled convection of heat carried by the blood stream.

Both conduction and convection obey the same form of linearity law which has been enunciated for all the transfers considered in the previous chapters: flow is proportional to the force generating it. In this case heat flow (H) across unit area of a conducting layer is proportional to the temperature difference (ΔT):

$$H = C \cdot \Delta T \tag{1}$$

The proportionality constant (C) is called the *thermal conductance*. It is the basic parameter used to describe heat flow by conduction-convection through all the layers of the skin; it normally includes both processes. Its unit is heat flow per unit area $\times$ temperature difference. Conductances in parallel are added linearly. Conductances in series are added by their reciprocals; the reciprocal of conductance is termed the *insulation* of the layer ($I = 1/C$), so that insulations in series are added linearly.

When a conducting layer may be considered uniform throughout its thickness (h) its specific conductance or thermal conductivity (k) may be derived:

$$k = hC$$

Conductivity is usually cited only when convection is absent; in the presence of convection it is termed "apparent" or "effective" conductivity. Conductivity is a measure of the behaviour of the material of which the conducting layer is composed, while conductance and insulation are measures of its effectiveness as a whole.

Blood Flow and Thermal Conduction

Blood flow across a tissue layer can be related to the change in conductance it produces (C_{blood}). If there is no exchange of heat between the blood and the tissue within the layer then:

$$C_{blood} = ms$$

where m = mass flow of blood (mass per unit area $\times$ time)

s = specific heat of blood

If some of the heat in the blood is exchanged with venous blood flowing back across the tissue layer then:

$$C_{blood} = \frac{ms}{1+\alpha} \tag{2}$$

where α is the countercurrent exchange factor, dependent itself on the conductance between the artery and vein and on the mass flow (cf. Appendix VI for derivation of equation 2).

The increase of conductivity due to the blood flow (k_{blood}) is dependent on the thickness of the layer through which this equation applies:

$$k_{\text{blood}} = \frac{msh}{1+\alpha} \tag{3}$$

and is therefore not easily related theoretically to the blood flow itself.

Units

Heat flow has been measured in three units by different observers (kcal/m²h; kcal/m²24 h; mcal/cm²sec) and units of conductance, insulation and conductivity have been derived from each of these units. The unit mcal/cm² is used uniformly throughout the present description, so that conductance is expressed in mcal/cm²sec°C, insulation in cm²sec°C/mcal, and conductivity in mcal/cm sec°C. The conversion factors used are listed below.

Conductance:

$$1 \text{ mcal/cm}^2\text{sec}°\text{C} = 36 \text{ kcal/m}^2\text{h}°\text{C}$$
$$= 864 \text{ kcal/m}^2\text{24 h}°\text{C}$$

Conductivity:

$$1 \text{ mcal/cm sec}°\text{C} = 36 \text{ kcal cm/m}^2\text{h}°\text{C*}$$
$$= 864 \text{ kcal cm/m}^2\text{24 h}°\text{C*}$$

Insulation:

$$1 \text{ cm}^2\text{sec}°\text{C/mcal} = 0.0278 \text{ m}^2\text{h}°\text{C/kcal}$$
$$= 0·00116 \text{ m}^2\text{24 h}°\text{C/kcal}$$
$$= 0·154 \text{ clo units}$$

The "clo" unit is an arbitrary unit, originally defined as equal to the insulation of a standard business suit (Burton and Edholm, 1955). It has been widely employed.

METHODS

Two measurements are required to define the conductance of a layer, the temperature difference across it, and the heat flow through it (equation 1). The following paragraphs describe the principal difficulties inherent in these measurements, and the ways in which they may be overcome.

* These two are "bastard" units containing both metre and cm units.

Temperature

The main difficulty in measuring temperature is the avoidance of heat flow along the measuring instrument, which would result in a change of temperature of the thermosensitive element. Two methods have been used to overcome this heat flow. In the first, the connexion to the thermosensitive element

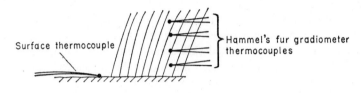

A   Connexion parallel to the skin surface

Surface thermocouple

Hammel's fur gradiometer thermocouples

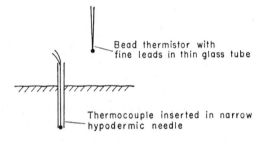

B   Low-conductance connexion

Bead thermistor with fine leads in thin glass tube

Thermocouple inserted in narrow hypodermic needle

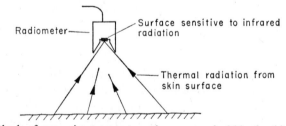

C   Surface radiation measurement

Radiometer

Surface sensitive to infrared radiation

Thermal radiation from skin surface

FIG. 53. Methods of measuring temperature above, on and within the skin.

is made along an isothermal plane, in this case parallel to the skin surface (Fig. 53A). Thus the connexion has a high conductance without inducing a great heat flow. This method has been used within fur *in vitro* (Hammel, 1955) and is the common means for measuring skin surface temperatures (for a detailed description of the calibration and design of surface thermometers, see Molnar and Rosenbaum, 1963).

The second method is to reduce the conductance of the connexion so that it is negligible relative to the conductance between the thermosensitive element and the surrounding tissue or air (Fig. 53B). Since metals have a very high conductivity relative to liquids and gases it is very difficult to ensure this. Nevertheless practical tests have shown that it can be done, either in air (Tregear, 1965a) or within tissue. It is the only practical method of measuring temperature gradients within living skin, and has been widely employed (e.g. Pennes, 1949; Reader, 1952; Irving, 1956; Irving and Hart, 1957).

A third method which has been used to measure transient changes in skin surface temperatures over limited skin areas is the measurement of thermal radiation (Fig. 53C). This is an accurate and sophisticated technique (Lipkin and Hardy, 1954) but too complex for general use.

Heat Flow

The main difficulty in measuring heat flow is the absence of perfect thermal insulators; the natural insulators of fat and fur are as good as the artificial ones out of which apparatus can be constructed. Thus the avoidance of heat leaks is a difficult problem. Three forms of direct calorimeter are in general use.

Absolute calorimetry

In this method a known amount of heat is supplied to one surface of the tissue electrically. Heat loss except through the tissue is reduced by guarding the other directions with surfaces maintained at the same temperature as the electrically heated block (Fig. 54A). Such devices have been widely used to measure the conductance of tissue and fur *in vitro* (Roeder, 1934; Scholander *et al.*, 1950a; Hammel, 1955; Tregear, 1965a). The method is absolute in that it does not depend on prior knowledge of conductivity in other insulators.

Gradient layer calorimetry

In this method the tissue layer is placed in series with an insulating layer whose conductance is known (Fig. 54B). The heat input into the system is not measured directly, but may be calculated from the temperature drop across the calibrated insulator, according to equation 1. The method has been further refined by the use of calibrated insulators which are themselves thermoelectric generators, i.e. they produce a voltage proportional to the temperature drop across them (Hatfield, 1950; Lentz and Hart, 1960).

The gradient layer principle has been applied to the measurement of heat flow through tissue layers and fur *in vitro* (Hatfield and Pugh, 1951; Hatfield, 1953; Lentz and Hart, 1960), and through small areas of living skin (Hatfield,

1950; Reader, 1952). It has also been used to measure heat loss from the finger (Burton and Edwards, 1960a), hand (Forster *et al.*, 1946), foot (Love, 1949) or the whole body (Benzinger and Kitzinger, 1949).

Comparative surface calorimetry

In this method heat is passed into the surface of living skin and the resultant temperature gradient along the surface of the skin is measured (Fig. 54C). As the conductivity of the surface layers of the skin alters, due to

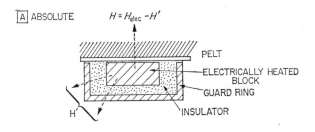

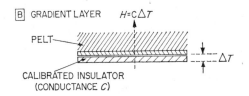

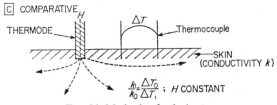

FIG. 54. Methods of calorimetry.

changes in blood flow, the temperature drop along the surface varies inversely. The apparatus can be calibrated on insulators of known conductivity. The purpose of these devices is to measure blood flow; they have been used successfully in body regions where the blood flow changes are great (Hensel and Bender, 1956; Aschoff and Wever, 1959).

Indirect calorimetry

The total heat production by an animal may be computed from its oxygen uptake (see Blaxter (1962) for details of the methods involved). In heat

balance this production is equal to its heat loss so that when various allow-
ances have been made the heat loss through the skin may be obtained. Under
conditions where this loss is expected to take place evenly over the whole
surface the heat loss per unit area may be calculated. This method has been
widely employed for the estimation of heat losses of animals in a cold environment (Scholander *et al.*, 1950a-c; Irving and Hart, 1957; Blaxter, 1962).

CONDUCTION AND RADIATION THROUGH AIR

The outermost insulative layer around the body is the still air which coats
the outside of the fur or naked skin. All surfaces exert a drag on the air above

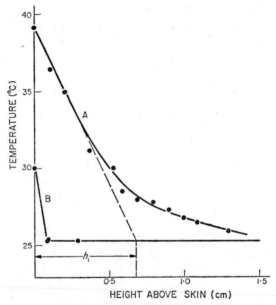

FIG. 55. The temperature profile above shaved skin in the absence of wind (A) and in a
wind of 8 miles/h (B). The effective still air thickness in the absence of wind has been constructed (h_1). (From Tregear, 1965a.)

them and so have a layer of truly still air in contact with them. Above this the
air becomes progressively more stirred. This can be seen by the temperature
gradient above warm, naked skin *in vitro* in the absence of wind (line A,
Fig. 55). The gradient is steepest near the skin where the air is still and therefore of lowest effective conductivity. As one proceeds away from the skin the
gradient progressively flattens, until above 1·5 cm it tends asymptotically
towards the general air temperature. In a wind the still air layer is much
thinner, and its edge is more distinct (line B, Fig. 55); once the drag of the
skin has been overcome the conductivity of the air is effectively infinite.

In order to describe the insulative effect of free air above a surface one may define an "effective" still air layer, which is the layer of truly still air which would cause the same insulation as the progressively more stirred layers actually do (h_1 in Fig. 55). The conductance of the air due to *conduction-convection* (C'_{air}) is therefore

$$C'_{air} = \frac{k_{air}}{h_1} \tag{4}$$

$$k_{air} = 0 \cdot 055 \text{ mcal/cm sec}°\text{C}$$

Since air is transparent to radiation the exchange of thermal radiation with the radiant environment is in parallel with the conductive exchange. As long as the radiant environment is at the same temperature as the air, the radiant exchange is equivalent to a thermal conductance (C_R) of approximately $0 \cdot 15$ mcal/cm^{2}sec$°$C (Appendix VII). The total conductance of the free air layer over skin (C'_{air}) is therefore

$$C_{air} = C'_{air} + C_R \beta$$

$$= \frac{0 \cdot 055}{h_1} + 0 \cdot 15 \, \beta \tag{5}$$

where β is the proportion of the surface area which is available for radiation.

For excised skin $\beta = 1 \cdot 0$; for the general body surface β is less than unity because some of the skin faces other skin and therefore exchanges less radiation with the external environment. For man $\beta = 0 \cdot 65 – 0 \cdot 77$, dependent on posture (Gagge *et al.*, 1938; Guibert and Taylor, 1952). No direct measurements have been made on animals, and a figure of $0 \cdot 7$ is usually assumed (Blaxter, 1962).

Solar radiation is quite separate from the thermal radiation exchange. It is, of course, independent of the temperature of the skin or the air, and therefore cannot be considered in terms of conductance. It represents a heat flow of up to 20 mcal/cm^{2}sec through the still air into the surface of the fur or naked skin (cf. Chapter 4).

In the absence of wind, the effective still air layer thickness (h_1) is dependent on the degree of thermal convection present, which is in turn dependent on the temperature difference between the skin and the air, and on the size and orientation of the exposed skin surface. If the heated, lighter air is free to move upwards, it creates convection currents (Gates, 1962). Over a plane surface several cm in diameter and 15$°$ C above the ambient air h_1 was found to be up to $0 \cdot 7$ cm thick (Fig. 55). Such a still air layer produces a conductance of $0 \cdot 1 – 0 \cdot 2$ mcal/cm^{2}sec$°$C (Siple and Passel, 1945; Tregear, 1965a) in parallel with the radiative conductance of $0 \cdot 15$ mcal/cm^{2}sec$°$C. The radiative heat flow from the surface of a mammal is therefore expected to be similar to the convective flow in the absence of wind. For men Gagge *et al.* (1938) found directly that the two losses were equal. Indirect calorimetry on other species indicates that more than half the heat loss occurs by radiation; the effective still air layer, calculated from equation 5, is 0·5–0·9 cm thick (Table XIX).

TABLE XIX. *Thermal conductance of still free air over skin, derived from whole-body calorimetry*
The net thermal conductance, including radiation, is given (C_{air}) and the thickness of the effective still air layer (h_1) calculated on equation 5, with $\beta = 0.7$.

Species	C_{air} (mcal/cm²sec°C)	h_1 (cm)	Reference
Man	0·22	0·5	Gagge *et al.* (1938)
Sheep	0·16	0·9	
Calf	0·20	0·5	Blaxter (1962)
Steer	0·19	0·6	
Pig, newborn	0·20	0·5	Mount (1959)
Guinea-pig	0·17	0·8	
Rat	0·18	0·7	Herrington (1940)
Mouse	0·19	0·6	

Once a mild wind blows most of the still air layer is stripped off the skin (Fig. 55). A wind of 2 miles/h more than doubles the heat loss from a 10 cm diameter cylinder (Hardy, 1949), which represents a trebling of the *conductive* conductance and reduction of h_1 to less than 0·3 cm. Higher wind speeds continue to reduce h_1 and increase conductance; physical experiments show that the conductance over a surface is approximately proportional to the square root of the wind velocity. For a cylinder 1·8 cm in diameter

$$C_{air} = 0.27 + 0.49 v^{0.5} \qquad (6; \text{Gold}, 1935)$$

where v = wind speed (m/sec)

The exact value of the proportionality constant in this equation depends on the size and shape of the surface. Nevertheless, the main conclusions are simple: in a wind speed of 5 miles/h or above the still air layer over skin is reduced to 0·2 cm or less, nearly all the heat is lost by convection rather than radiation, and the conductance of the free air becomes so high that in most instances its insulation is small relative to that of the other layers below it.

Thus under optimum conditions the still air above an animal's fur or skin is a considerable insulator, limited mainly by the radiation through it, but it is a very fragile barrier, easily destroyed by movement of the air or the body.

CONDUCTION THROUGH FUR

A great deal of work has been done on the mechanism of hair growth, notably in the rodents and the sheep. The types and structural features of hair have been classified (Dry, 1925, 1928; Wildman, 1954; Ramanathan et al., 1955), the growth cycles of various species have been described (Ryder, 1964; Side and Rudall, 1964) and the cellular and biochemical mechanisms of growth elucidated (Ryder, 1955; Rudall and Durward, 1958; Ebling, 1964). For the present purpose, however, this work is largely irrelevant. Only two parameters are known to influence thermal conduction through fur, the total thickness of the pelt (h_2) and the hair density. Fur is commonly 0·5–8 cm thick (Fig. 56) and its hair density varies from 10/cm^2, in the "physiologically naked" species, to 5 000/cm^2 in the most densely furred species (Table XX).

In the absence of wind, the thermal insulation of dense fur is proportional to its thickness (Fig. 56), i.e. its conductivity (k_{fur}) is uniform throughout its depth

$$C_{fur} = \frac{k_{fur}}{h_2} \tag{7}$$

The conductivity of fur has been estimated from experiments on excised skin by various observers, according to equation 7 (Table XXI). The values vary between 0·09 and 0·12 mcal/cm sec°C, 1·5–2 × the conductivity of truly still air and equal to the conductivity of many commercial air-filled insulators. The conductivity is much lower than that of most solid insulators (Table XXI). Hammel (1955) showed that the conductance of dense fur was reduced by three-quarters when the air within the fur was replaced by Freon, a denser, less conductive gas. Thus at least three-quarters of the conductance through fur is via the air itself and not through the hairs. Furthermore Finck (1930) showed that conduction in the fibres of an air-filled insulator only became important when more than 20% of the volume was taken up by the solid, and even in the densest furs calculation shows that < 10% of the volume is hair.

Nevertheless, the apparent conductivity of dense fur is considerably greater than that of still air. Part of the extra heat loss is probably due to evaporation through the fur (Hammel, 1955), and part is due to convection, which is almost impossible to eradicate completely within insulators (Finck, 1930; Hammel, 1955; Burton and Edholm, 1955). Such convection is not critically dependent on the orientation of the surface, for the conductance of dense fur is not greatly affected by inverting the pelt (Lentz and Hart, 1960).

In furs of low density, where the skin is visible between the hairs, radiation loss must also occur. Radiative loss through artificial insulators becomes important when < 2% of the volume is filled by the solid (Finck, 1930; Pratt, 1962). In dense fur, radiation exchange is negligible (Hammel, 1955).

The effect of wind on conduction through fur has been comparatively little studied, which is surprising since the obvious function of fur is to retain air in a wind. Lentz and Hart (1960) demonstrated how well dense fur fulfils this function; a 35 miles/h wind was needed to double the heat loss through an excised caribou pelt, compared to the 2 miles/h needed over a naked

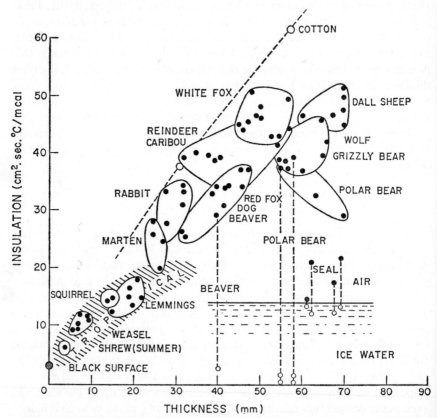

Fig. 56. Insulation in relation to winter fur thickness in a series of Arctic mammals. The insulation in tropical mammals is indicated by the shaded area. In the aquatic mammals (seal, beaver, polar bear) the measurements in 0° C air are connected by vertical broken lines with the same measurements taken in ice water. In all cases the hot plate guard ring unit was kept at 37° C and the outside air or water at 0° C. The two upper points of the lemmings are from *Dicrostonyx*, the others from *Lemmus*. (Redrawn from Scholander *et al.*, 1950a.)

surface (Hardy, 1949). The insulation of the fur was affected by the wind only a little more than that of a fixed insulator. The direction of the wind relative to the natural lie of the fur had little effect on the relationship of insulation to wind speed, but wind blown directly at the pelt reduced the insulation more than wind blowing past it. Bennett and Hutchinson (1964) found that a 10 miles/h wind had only a slight effect on the insulation of dense Merino sheep fur.

Tregear (1965a) studied the effect of hair density on the insulation of fur in a wind. Dense rabbit fur (5 000 hairs/cm^2) was as insensitive to wind as

TABLE XX. *Hair density on the general body surface of various mammals*

Species	Hair density (hairs/cm^2 skin)	Reference
Man, torso	60	Szabo (1962)
leg	50	
Pig, flank	40	
belly	10	
Horse, flank	1 300	Tregear (1965a)*
belly	800	
Cow	600–2 000	Dowling (1956)
Sheep	800–5 000	Carter and Clarke (1957)
Rabbit, back	4 000	Tregear (1965a)*
Caribou	2 600–5 000	Lentz and Hart (1960)

* These figures are derived from a small number of specimens; variations such as those found by the other authors are also to be expected in these species.

TABLE XXI. *Thermal conductivity of some biological and physical insulators*

Material	k (mcal/cm sec°C)	Reference
Air	0·055	Washburn (1929)
Rabbit fur	0·09	Tregear (1965a)
Arctic mammal fur	0·10	Hart (1956)
	0·12	Scholander et al. (1950a)
	0·09	Hammel (1955)
Merino sheep fur	0·10	Bennett and Hutchinson (1964)
Cotton wool	0·10	Gray (1963)
Nylon pile	0·11	Hammel (1955)
Jute	0·09	Finck (1930)
Mineral wool	0·10	Gray (1963)
Wool	0·10	
Polystyrenes	0·1–0·4	Bernhardt (1959)
Polyethylene	0·8	
Polyvinyls	0·3–0·5	
Rubber	0·52	Hatfield (1953)

Lentz and Hart's caribou fur. The insulation of horse hair (1 000/cm^2) was halved by an 8 miles/h wind, whilst that of pigs (40/cm^2) was reduced to one-seventh of its original value. However, even the sparse hair of pigs considerably increased the drag of the skin on the air: the conductance of the air over

G

shaved pig skin in an 8 miles/h wind was more than double that over unshaved skin.

The most illuminating point to emerge from this work was that the temperature within the wind-blown fur fell linearly from the skin surface to some point within the fur, where it reached that of the ambient air (Fig. 57). Thus the conductivity within the lower part of the fur was uniform, and

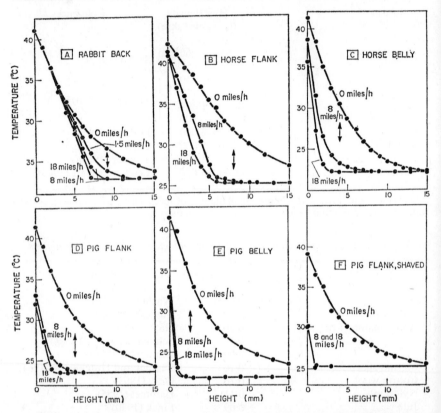

Fig. 57. Temperature gradient above the skin surface through furs of different species, and exposed to various wind speeds. The upper surface of the fur is indicated by a vertical arrow. The temperatures were registered on a fine bead thermistor. (Tregear, 1965a.)

calculation showed that in the denser furs it was unaffected by wind speed. From this it may be deduced that the action of the wind is to bite into the fur to a certain depth, destroying entirely the insulation above that depth, but leaving the lower part of the fur unaffected.

The depth of fur which is stirred depends both on the hair density of the pelt, and on the wind speed (Fig. 58). More detailed work would be required to work out the exact relationship between these variables, but it is evident that the depth stirred is proportional to a power of the wind speed much less than unity (Fig. 57A) and that a hair density of 5 000/cm² will keep out most normal terrestrial winds, while a hair density of 1 000/cm² will not. This latter point is of particular importance, since several species have a hair density around 1 000/cm² (Table XX).

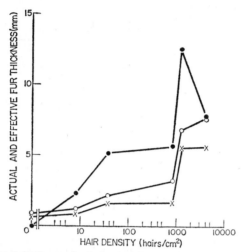

Fig. 58. The actual thickness of pelt from various species (●) and their effective thickness *in vitro* deduced from the temperature gradients within them in a wind of 8 miles/h (○) or of 18 miles/h (×). (From Tregear, 1965a.)

In summary, the fur acts as enclosed air, the upper layers of which are blown away by a wind. The behaviour of fur in still air has been adequately studied, but its behaviour in a wind has not.

CONDUCTION AND VASCULAR CONVECTION THROUGH SKIN

All liquids, and nearly all solids, conduct heat much faster than still air. The skin is therefore a much less efficient insulator, per unit thickness, than the fur. Nevertheless, when the fur is sparse and the skin is thick it can be the major insulation of the body.

The thermal conductivity of excised skin layers has been measured by many observers, using a variety of methods, over many decades; only the more reliable and recent observations are shown in Table XXII. All these authors except Lipkin and Hardy (1954) used the classical calorimetric methods described above. Lipkin and Hardy employed the thermal pulse technique, in which the temperature of the skin is measured during the application of a pulse of radiant heat to the surface (p. 118). The low value of muscle conductivity found by Hardy and Soderstrom (1938) has since been attributed to dehydration of the tissue (Hatfield and Pugh, 1951) and may be discounted. A series of values obtained by Ponder (1961) have not been included because they differ greatly from those of other workers, and were in several cases greatly above the conductivity of water.

From these results it appears that excised dermis is 1·5–1·8 × as conductive

TABLE XXII. *Thermal conductivity of some common liquids, of excised tissue and of tissue in vivo in the absence of blood flow*
All data refer to human material except where otherwise stated.

Material	k (mcal/cm sec°C)	Reference
Liquids		
Water	1·47	Washburn (1929)
Glycerol	0·68	
Olive oil	0·40	
Excised tissue		
Epidermis	0·50	Henriques and Moritz (1947a)
Dermis	0·70	Roeder (1934)
	0·90	Henriques and Moritz (1947a)
	0·77	Lipkin and Hardy (1954)
Fat	0·49	Hardy and Soderstrom (1938)
	0·40	Henriques and Moritz (1947a)
	0·49	Hatfield and Pugh (1951)
	0·52	Lipkin and Hardy (1954)
(bovine)	0·52	Hatfield (1953)
Muscle	1·00	Breuer (1924)
	0·47	Hardy and Soderstrom (1938)
	1·10	Henriques and Moritz (1947a)
	0·92	Hatfield and Pugh (1951)
	0·97	Lipkin and Hardy (1954)
(bovine)	1·27	Hatfield (1953)
Tissue *in vivo* without blood flow		
Skin	0·80	Aschoff and Kaempffer (1947)
	0·75	Reader (1952)
	0·90	Lipkin and Hardy (1954)
	0·70	Hensel and Bender (1956)
Fat	0·5–0·9	Daniels and Baker (1961)*
(seal)	0·5–0·7	Irving and Hart (1959)*
Muscle	1·27	Reader (1952)

* Without blood stasis, but in a cold environment, and therefore with minimal blood flow.

as fat, and that both are less conductive than muscle. The probable physical basis of this is that heat conduction through dermis and muscle is via the water molecules, while conduction through the fat is via the fat molecules, which are larger and of lower conductivity (Table XXII). It follows from this that the conductivity of connective tissue *in vivo* should vary quite widely with its water content; the quoted values for human dermis might, for instance, be far too high to apply to the dense dermis of pachyderms (Fig. 39.

Chapter 3). White fat, on the other hand, is of relatively uniform consistency (Barrnett, 1962; Chalmers, 1964) and would therefore be expected to have a similarly uniform conductivity. Although the dry layers of epidermis are less conductive than dermis (Table XXII), the epidermis is too thin to provide appreciable insulation. Its conductance is only important in the consideration of pulsatile applications of heat or cold leading to pain and burns or frostbite.

Measurements of thermal conductivity of tissues *in vivo* in the absence of blood flow have confirmed the results from excised tissue (Table XXII). The superficial layers of the skin have a conductivity of 0·7–0·9 mcal/cm sec°C, and muscle has a higher conductivity. The quoted values for fat were obtained indirectly from measurements of metabolic rate, and are therefore less accurate; there was some blood flowing through the fat in these experiments, which may account for the occasional high values obtained.

The net insulation provided by these layers has been measured in man under cold stress. It varies widely, but the average value obtained is approx. 5 cm^{2}sec°C/mcal (Benzinger, 1959; Hertzmann, 1961) equivalent to 3·5 cm of mixed fat and connective tissue. In species which have thick layers of subcutaneous fat, the insulation is 2–3 × as great as this (Irving, 1956; Irving and Hart, 1957).

Blood Flow and Heat Convection in the Skin

Most of the blood vessels of human skin terminate near to the epidermis (Ellis, 1961) and in the skin of the extremities there are specialized arteriovenous anastamoses to regulate the blood flow (Welbourn, 1964). The human cutaneous circulation is highly dependent on the thermal balance of the subject; in the cold it is usually less than 0·02 ml/cm^{2}min, whilst under heat stress it can rise to 0·3 ml/cm^{2}min (Hertzmann and Randall, 1948), although it is more usually 0·05 ml/cm^{2}min (Hertzmann, 1953). Thus in man under heat stress the skin circulation is grossly in excess of that required to supply the tissue with metabolites and oxygen. This high blood flow increases the thermal conductance of the skin from its minimal value of 0·2 mcal/cm^{2}sec°C to 1·2 mcal/cm^{2}sec°C, or occasionally much higher values (Hertzmann, 1961; Benzinger, 1959). Thus a blood flow of 1 μl/cm^{2}sec (0·06 ml/cm^{2}min) produces a skin conductance of 1 mcal/cm^{2}sec°C. This is in accordance with theory; in equation 2, if $\alpha = 0$ and $s = 1$, $C_{blood} = m$, so that 1 μl/cm^{2}sec is equivalent to 1 mcal/cm^{2}sec°C. The thermal conductivity of the superficial tissues of the skin also rises under heat stress, by 1–3 mcal/cm sec°C (Lipkin and Hardy, 1954). If the blood flow in these experiments was similar to that measured by Hertzmann, then again the conductivity change may be theoretically related to the blood flow. In equation 3, if $\alpha = 0$ and $s = 1$, $k_{blood} = mh$. According to the measurements under cold stress (see previous section)

$h = 3\cdot5$ cm, so that a blood flow of 1 μl/cm^{2}sec should produce a conductivity change of $3\cdot5$ mcal/cm sec$^\circ$C. The actual change seen is somewhat smaller, but considering the number of assumptions involved, the agreement is remarkably good.

The other experiments in which thermal conductivity was related to blood flow were performed on the finger (Hensel and Bender, 1956; Aschoff and Wever, 1959) where the vascular convection is past the skin, not into it. They are therefore not directly comparable to Hertzmann and Lipkin and Hardy's results.

All the above results refer to human skin. Exposed surfaces on other mammals also contain a circulation which responds to heat stress: this has been proven in the rabbit's ear (Grant, 1935), the monkey's tail (Hongo and Luck, 1953), the seal's flipper (Irving and Hart, 1957) and the stork's leg (Kahl, 1963), and may be a general function of all physiologically naked skin. Under fur the cutaneous blood supply is related primarily to the nutrition of the hair follicle (Rudall and Durward, 1958; Ryder, 1955) and does not appear to be increased by thermal stress (Hammel et al., 1958).

In summary, the insulation of human skin can be cut down very sharply by the cutaneous circulation, to less than 1 cm^{2}sec$^\circ$C/mcal, and this reduction can be related theoretically to the blood flow. Exposed areas of other mammals possess the same faculty, but fur-covered areas do not.

VASCULAR CONVECTION AND COUNTERCURRENT EXCHANGE IN LIMBS

The limb of a mammal under cold stress is often cooler than the central body, so that the whole limb acts as an insulator (Pennes, 1949). The insulation of a limb in the absence of blood flow is dependent on its passive conduction. As the tissues of the body have conductivities lower than that of water (Table XXII) the insulation provided by a limb which is considerably longer than it is wide is much greater when its core temperature is allowed to fall, and this can be of great advantage to an animal under cold stress. The melting points of the fats within the limb are lower than those in the torso, so that they do not freeze when the temperature falls (Schmidt-Nielsen, 1946; Irving et al., 1957). However, the tissues of the limb require blood for their metabolism, and this blood is bound to carry heat with it.

Heat loss due to blood flow is reduced when the outgoing arterial blood exchanges heat with the returning venous blood. For such a system to be efficient, the artery and vein must run alongside each other for a considerable length; the situation is expressed mathematically in Appendix VI. In fact, arteries and veins leading to limbs often do run alongside one another. In the porpoise, the arteries which supply the exposed fins and flukes are each surrounded by a ring of veins (Scholander and Schevill, 1955). In sloths, anteaters, lemurs and storks the main artery supplying the limb breaks up into many small branches, each accompanied by two small veins, and proceeds along the limb as a rete of blood vessels (Wislocki, 1928; Wislocki and Straus, 1932; Wislocki and Enders, 1935; Barnett *et al.*, 1958; Kahl, 1963). Such retia are also found in aquatic mammals such as the manatee, porpoise and seal (Fawcett, 1942; Barnett *et al.*, 1958). Even where these specialized systems are absent, it is usual to find that each artery is accompanied by a vein or veins (Brück and Hensel, 1953). The anatomical basis for countercurrent heat exchange is therefore present in all limbs and is highly developed in some species.

The efficacy of the heat exchange has been demonstrated directly in the sloth (Scholander and Krog, 1957) and man (Bazett *et al.*, 1949; Brück and Hensel, 1953) by the extremely steep temperature gradient along blood vessels through which there is a considerable flow of blood. Arteriovenous exchange may also be inferred from the steep temperature gradient along the upper parts of the legs of oxen (Whittow, 1962) and several species of Arctic mammal (Irving and Krog, 1954) in the presence of continued blood flow. There is also a steep temperature gradient along the flippers of cold-stressed seals (Irving and Hart, 1957) and the legs of cold-stressed armadillos (Johanssen, 1961).

The most extreme examples of countercurrent exchange are found among the wading and swimming birds. Scholander (1955) showed that the Arctic gull lost only a few per cent more heat when its legs were placed in ice-cold water, although its web was supplied with blood, and Kahl (1963) has demonstrated the efficiency of the upper-leg rete in the wood stork.

These countercurrent systems may be by-passed under heat stress by the use of an alternative venous return.

EVAPORATION

Evaporation from the skin surface is in parallel with conduction through the fur and still air above it. As water has a high latent heat of vaporization ($L = 580$ cal/g at 30° C; Hodgman, 1963), it is a potent means of increasing heat loss under heat stress, while the impermeability of the epidermis is sufficient to make the obligatory heat loss by cutaneous evaporation small relative to the animal's basal metabolism.

PRODUCTION OF WATER ON THE SKIN SURFACE

The human insensible water loss, the water loss through skin in the absence of active sweating, is usually in the region of 20 μg/cm^{2}min, although different estimates have given widely different results (Table IIIA, p. 8).

This evaporation rate (E) is equivalent to a heat loss (H_e) of $0\cdot2$ mcal/cm^{2}sec, $(H_e = LE)$ which is approximately one-fifth of the basal metabolic rate of man (cf. Table XXIV, p. 138). It is thus a small, but not a negligible, part of the heat loss from the body. This obligatory water loss can be supplemented by sweat under conditions of heat stress. Nearly all mammalian skin contains sweat glands; the most notable exception is the hairy skin of the rodent. The sweat glands have been extensively studied, and the description which follows is only a brief summary of those findings which are most relevant to thermal function.

Human Eccrine Sweat Glands

The whole body surface of man is supplied by a high density of coiled tubular sweat glands. Their numbers vary from 100 to 600/cm^2 (Szabo, 1962); the highest density is found in the palms, soles, cheek and forehead. The structure and biochemistry of these glands have been exhaustively investigated (Montagna, 1962; Montagna et al., 1962). On nervous or hormonal stimulation they secrete an aqueous solution, nearly free of electrolytes when the secretion rate is slow, but approximating to the osmotic pressure of blood during high and prolonged sweating (Robinson and Robinson, 1954). When stimulation ceases they can reabsorb some of their secretion (Thompson, 1962).

Under thermal stress the maximum rate of water production by these glands is 2–3 mg/cm^{2}min (Table XXIII). A rate of 1–1·5 mg/cm^{2}min can be maintained for long periods, representing a heat loss of 10–15 mcal/cm^{2}sec. Repeated application of heat stress increases the steady sweat rate which can be produced (Conn, 1949; Fox et al., 1964). If the sweat does not all evaporate the glands may become blocked and further sweat production impaired (Shelley, 1954).

The human apocrine sweat glands are not primarily thermal in function (Hurley and Shelley, 1960).

Sweat Glands of the Friction Surfaces in other Mammals

Eccrine sweat glands have been found in the foot pads of all those mammals which have been examined, including the rodents (Marzulli and Callahan, 1957; Montagna, 1962) and on the flippers of seals (Bartholomew and Wilke, 1956). The glands of the cat's foot pad have been used as a model system in which to examine the mechanism of reabsorption of sweat (Lloyd, 1960, 1962). The main function of these glands appears to be mechanical, in moistening the frictional surfaces (Montagna, 1962), but the glands of some species do respond to thermal stress (Marzulli and Callahan, 1957).

Glands of the General Body Surface in Mammals other than Man

Most mammals have sweat glands on their general body surface. Their presence has been definitely established in the monkey (Marzulli and Callahan, 1957; Montagna, 1962), sloth (Wislocki, 1928), dog (Dempsey, 1946), cat (Marzulli and Callahan, 1957), sheep (Brook and Short, 1960), cow (Dempsey,

TABLE XXIII. *Maximal production of sweat on the body surface of various species under thermal stress*
These measurements were obtained either by a capsule technique or by the total cutaneous water loss from the animal.

Species	Sweat rate $(mg/cm^2 min)$	Reference
Man		
(a) For short periods	2·2	Moss (1923)
	2·5	Eichna *et al.* (1945)
	3·0	Ladell (1945)
(b) For period of several hours	1·0–1·5	Robinson and Gerking (1947)
	1·4	Moss (1923)
Cow	0·2–0·3	Kibler and Brody (1952)
	0·5–1·0	McDowell *et al.* (1954)
	1·0	Ferguson and Dowling (1956)
Sheep	0·1	Knapp and Robinson (1954)
	0·05	Brook and Short (1960)
	0·04	Alexander and Williams (1962)
Dog	0·1	Hammel *et al.* (1958)
Donkey	0·6	Schmidt-Nielsen *et al.* (1957)
Camel	0·4	Schmidt-Nielsen *et al.* (1957)

1946), pig (Mount, 1962), hippopotamus (Luck and Wright, 1959), horse (Marzulli and Callahan, 1957), donkey and camel (Schmidt-Nielsen *et al.*, 1957). They are definitely absent in rodents and rabbits (Marzulli and Callahan, 1957). These glands have generally been termed apocrine because of their resemblance to human apocrine glands and their common, but not invariant, association with hair follicles (Montagna, 1962). However, at least in the cow their secretion is not necrobiotic (Findlay and Jenkinson, 1960).

Although most species have sweat glands all over their skin many appear not to use them in heat stress. Thus, although the dog's sweat glands can be activated chemically (Aoki, 1955), their response to thermal stress is slight and ineffective (Marzulli and Callahan, 1957; Hammel *et al.*, 1958). Cats do not appear to sweat under thermal stress (Prouty, 1949; Marzulli and Callahan, 1957) nor do pigs (Mount, 1965). Sweating in sheep can sometimes be produced by thermal stress (Cragg and Davies, 1947; Alexander and Williams,

G*

1962) and sometimes not (Knapp and Robinson, 1954). Even when it does occur, the secretion rate is low (Table XXIII) and has little effect on the heat balance of the animal (Blaxter et al., 1959).

On the other hand, heat stress causes sweating over the general body surface at thermally significant rates in donkeys, camels and cows (Table XXIII), and probably also does so in horses and burros (Marzulli and Callahan, 1957).

EVAPORATION OF WATER FROM THE SKIN

Principles

As long as the supply of heat to a wetted surface is sufficient to maintain its temperature constant, the evaporation from the surface is proportional to the difference in vapour concentration between the air at the skin surface and the ambient air:

$$E = \frac{D}{h_0}(q_s - q_a) \tag{8}$$

where D = diffusivity of water in air ($D = 0.24$ cm^2/sec; Hodgman, 1963)

h_0 = effective still air layer over the skin, including air in the fur

q_s = vapour concentration at skin surface

q_a = vapour concentration in ambient air

The vapour concentration in the ambient air is determined by the relative humidity (r_a) and the concentration of saturated water vapour at the temperature of the air (Q_a); $q_a = r_a Q_a$. The saturated vapour concentration is highly dependent on temperature (Fig. 59) so that in cold air the vapour concentration gradient between skin and air is always large, and is little dependent on the relative humidity. When the ambient air temperature approaches that of the skin, on the other hand, the vapour concentration gradient is critically dependent on the relative humidity.

The vapour concentration at the skin surface is not directly measurable. If the skin is completely wet, then it is equal to the saturated vapour concentration at the skin surface temperature ($q_s = Q_s$). However, this is an extreme case, and rarely seen. In general, the vapour concentration is less than the saturated value. One may define a parameter, called the relative humidity of the skin surface (r_s), such that $q_s = r_s Q_s$ (Mole, 1948). On this definition equation 8 becomes

$$E = \frac{D}{h_0}(r_s Q_s - r_a Q_a) \tag{9a}$$

However, it must be emphasized that r_s is an empirical parameter which is calculated from the experimental measurements, not a means of prediction.

An alternative parameter to the surface relation humidity is the "wetted fraction" (γ; Gagge, 1937). This concept supposes that a fraction γ of the skin is completely wet, and that the rest of the skin is dry, so that

$$E = \frac{\gamma D}{h_0}(Q_s - r_a Q_a) \tag{9b}$$

The concept of relative humidity is probably more realistic at low sweat rates, when the surface of the skin is not fully wetted, while wetted fraction may be used when a portion of the whole area is truly moist.

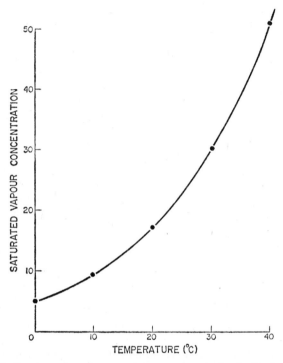

FIG. 59. Concentration of saturated water vapour ($\mu g/cm^3$). (Hodgman, 1963.)

If the vapour concentration difference between the skin and the ambient air is known, as when the skin is completely wet, the evaporation rate is dependent only on the effective still air layer. This layer includes the still air within and above the fur ($h_0 = h_1 + h_2$). If h_0 is several cm thick, even the maximum vapour concentration difference available, 45 $\mu g/cm^2$ when the skin is at 38° C and the ambient air is completely dry (Fig. 59), will not suffice to produce a thermally significant evaporation rate (Fig. 60). On the other hand, if $h_0 = 0 \cdot 1$ cm, then a modest vapour concentration difference will allow evaporation at the maximum rate which the sweat glands can produce.

Methods of Measuring Sweat Evaporation

Sweat loss from the skin can be measured in the same way as insensible water loss (Chapter 1) by weight loss of the body or by increase of vapour concentration within a capsule. It is much easier to measure than insensible water loss, because the mass of water concerned is much greater. The major

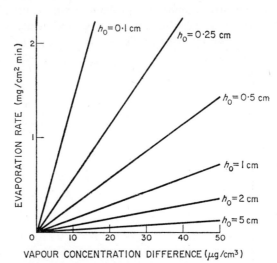

FIG. 60. Theoretical relationship (equation 9) between evaporation rate and concentration gradient for different thicknesses of still air (h_0).

difficulties in the measurement are the construction of a reliable humidity sensor, and the provision of conditions of airflow within the capsule similar to those outside it (McLean, 1963).

Practical Cases of Evaporation

The effective still air layer over human skin is approximately 0·6 cm in the absence of wind, and falls to 0·2 cm or less in the presence of a mild breeze (p. 122). It follows that a nude man should be able to evaporate all of the sweat he produces into dry air (Fig. 60), and in desert climates men wearing light, loose clothing do not show overt water on the skin, however high the heat stress (Adolph, 1947). Under steamy tropical conditions, however, the vapour concentration difference may drop to $10\,\mu g/cm^3$; at this point even 0·2 cm of still air presents a considerable resistance to evaporation, and an evaporation rate equal to the maximum steady sweat rate of $1·5\,\mu g/cm^2min$ cannot be maintained (Fig. 60). For nude man wind is always a strong aid to evaporation, because he has no fur to keep the value of h_0 high in spite of air movement.

Cows, camels and donkeys, the other animals whose sweat rate is reasonably accurately known, all have much denser hair than man, so that their effective still air layer is thicker, and cannot be so greatly reduced by a wind; as the pelt is usually 0·5–2 cm thick, h_0 will not fall below this value except in a strong wind. It follows that their possible evaporation rate, even in desert conditions, is lower than that of man (Fig. 60), and is in fact in the region of their maximal sweat production rates, 0·4–1 mg/cm² min. Clearly under steamy tropical conditions sweat production by an animal with 2 cm of fur would be of comparatively little thermal use (Fig. 60).

In many of the animals which are known not to sweat under heat stress the fur is too thick to allow thermally effective sweating, e.g. a white fox with 5 cm of dense fur could only evaporate 0·1 mg/cm²min into dry air. The pig, on the other hand, fails to sweat although its body surface is fully available for evaporation.

THE HEAT BALANCE OF THE ANIMAL

PRINCIPLES

The physical processes of heat loss through the skin have been described in the previous sections. Having analysed the thermal insulation, it can be re-synthesized to see how it accounts for the heat balance of the animal.

When an animal is in heat balance, its heat loss equals its heat gain, and so its deep body temperature remains constant. At rest, and in the absence of solar radiation, the heat gain of the body is the basal metabolic rate. The basal metabolic rate (H_{m_0}) of different species is proportional to a power of their body weight which is slightly greater than two-thirds (Kleiber, 1947), while their surface area is proportional to the two-thirds power exactly, for a given shape. It follows that larger mammals produce slightly more heat per unit area of skin surface than smaller ones; over the whole range of size from a 20 g mouse to a 4 000 kg elephant the variation is from 0·5 to 2·5 mcal/cm² sec (Table XXIV). There are large variations about this general law, of which the most notable are the high metabolic rates of the weasel and seal, and the low rates of the manatee and sloth.

The basal metabolic rate is in balance with heat loss at ambient temperatures down to a critical temperature below which the metabolic rate must be increased. Since the insulation (I_0) is constant below the critical temperature, in this range the metabolic rate (H_m) should be proportional to the temperature difference between the body and the air (T_b-T_a):

$$H_m = \frac{T_b - T_a}{I_0} \qquad (10)$$

This theoretical prediction has been shown to hold in practice for many species of mammal (Fig. 61). The critical temperature (T_c) is the point at which the line relating metabolic rate to air temperature strikes the basal

TABLE XXIV. *Basal metabolism of various species expressed as heat loss per unit area of skin surface (H_{m_0})*

Metabolic rates were obtained from (A) Kleiber (1947), (B) Scholander *et al.* (1950b), (C) Irving and Hart (1957) and (D) Blaxter (1962). The areas of the animals were deduced from their weights on the formula $A = kW^{2/3}$; $k = 0.10$ m²/kg²/³ (DuBois and DuBois, 1915).

Species	Weight (kg)	H_{m_0} (mcal/cm²sec)	Reference
Mouse	0·021	0·52	A
Lemming	0·050	0·88	B
Weasel	0·070	2·14	B
Rat	0·28	0·77	A
Guinea-pig	0·41	0·73	A
Night monkey	0·82	0·65	B
Rabbit	2·5	0·73	A
Cat	3·0	0·83	A
Two-toed sloth	3·8	0·34	B
White fox	4·7	1·47	B
Dog	14	1·02	A
Harbor seal	35	2·08	C
Sheep	46	1·46	D
Man	56	1·10	B
Porpoise	180	2·46	B
Manatee	250	0·83	B
Cow	480	2·30	D
Elephant	3 700	2·44	A

metabolism. T_c has been measured for many species (Fig. 61; Table XXV). The maximum insulation I_0 can be deduced from a knowledge of T_c and the basal metabolic rate:

$$I_0 = \frac{T_b - T_c}{H_{m_0}} \tag{11}$$

Values of I_0 calculated in this way are shown in the first column of Table XXVI.

Above the critical temperature the metabolic rate remains constant while the insulation falls until above a certain temperature heat balance can only be maintained by increased evaporation. I have termed this the "evaporation temperature" (T_e). In some species the extra evaporation is provided by panting, in some by salivation, and in others by sweating. The evaporation temperature is less clearly defined than the the the critical temperature, but some values derived from the literature are shown in Table XXV. At higher air temperatures than T_e the heat loss becomes dominated by evaporation, since the temperature difference between body and air is small. In this case the important parameter is the ambient vapour concentration, rather than the air

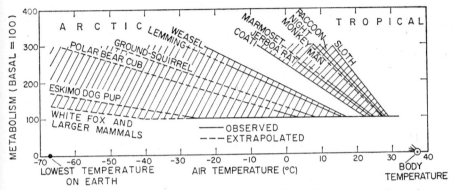

FIG. 61. The relation of metabolic rate ($H_{m_0} = 100\%$) to air temperature in various species. Note that the lines all point towards the body temperature, as predicted by equation 10. (From Scholander *et al.*, 1950c.)

temperature. When the maximum evaporation rate cannot balance the metabolic rate plus insolation, the deep body temperature starts to rise, and homoeothermy is lost.

HEAT BALANCE IN DENSELY FURRED MAMMALS

The critical temperatures of large Arctic mammals, who have a thick coat of dense fur, is extremely low. For the best-insulated species it is so low that Scholander *et al* (1950b, c) were unable to reach it under normal Arctic conditions (Fig. 61). Husky dogs can sleep happily without raising their metabolic rate in an Arctic gale at $-40°$ C. This confirms the great insulating power of dense fur and its impenetrability by wind. Moreover the insulation of these mammals deduced from their critical temperature and metabolism (I_0; equation 11) equals the measured insulation of their excised pelts (Table XXVI; value for white fox). Thus it appears that in these species under cold stress little heat is lost other than through the fur; probably the countercurrent exchange systems in the limbs are very efficient, particularly in the long-legged ungulates (Irving and Krog, 1954). The fur is the major insulation in the Arctic mammals; the temperature of the skin beneath it is near that of the deep body (Irving and Krog, 1954). In many species the fur thickness changes seasonally, so that in winter the insulation is increased and the critical temperature decreased (Irving *et al.*, 1955). Rain is a particular hazard to the fur's insulation; in young caribou it can be fatal (Hart *et al.*, 1961).

Other large mammals with thick dense fur are not so thermally efficient as the Arctic species. For instance, a sheep with a 5 cm fleece has theoretical fur insulation of 60 cm²sec°C/mcal but its critical temperature is only 10° C (Table XXV), equivalent to an insulation of 19 cm²sec°C/mcal (Table XXVI). Thus it must lose much of its heat through the thinly haired surface of its head and legs. Similarly the domestic dog has a very high critical temperature

TABLE XXV. *Critical temperature* (T_c) *and evaporation temperature* (T_e) *in various species under resting conditions*
The definitions of these two temperatures are given in the text.

Species	$T_c(°C)$	$T_e(°C)$	Reference
Densely furred			
Rat	26	29	Herrington (1940)
Mouse	25[1]	33[2]	Enger (1957)[1]; Herrington (1940)[2]
Guinea-pig	27	31	Herrington (1940)
Jerboa rat	25[1]	35[2]	Scholander *et al.* (1950c)[1]; Kirmiz (1962)[2]
Domestic dog	24	30	Hammel *et al.* (1958)
Husky dog	40	(>5)	Scholander *et al.* (1950b)
Sheep (5 cm fleece)	10	20	Blaxter *et al.* (1959)
Lightly furred			
Cow	7[1]	24[2]	Blaxter (1962)[1]; McLean (1963)[2]
Pig, newborn	31	33	Mount (1959, 1962)
adult	0	(>10)	Irving *et al.* (1956)
Man, nude	29	33	Gagge *et al.* (1938)
Aquatic			
Fur seal	0	—	Irving *et al.* (1962)
Harbor seal	10	—	Irving and Hart (1957)

The figures in parentheses are limits, based only on observation of the animals' behaviour. Superscript numbers refer to the references in column 4.

(Table XXV). The sloth, on the other hand, appears to use all its fur insulation effectively (Table XXVI) but its critical temperature is very high (Fig. 61) because its metabolic rate is abnormally low.

The small densely furred mammals also use their fur insulation efficiently, in that their overall insulation is approximately equal to that of their fur (Table XXVI). However, their fur is comparatively short so that its insulation is much less than that of the large animals and their critical temperatures are therefore very high (Table XXV). They survive in cold conditions by nest-building and burrowing, which provides extra insulation, and also by hibernation, in which their deep body temperature is allowed to drop to near that of the ambient air (Kayser, 1961).

The insulation of dense fur is invariant, and if it is much more than 1 cm thick evaporation through it cannot proceed at a thermally useful rate. In fact, thermal sweating through dense fur is only known in the sheep, where it occurs at a very low rate. Two avenues of heat loss under stress are open to the densely furred animal: it may expose its extremities for conduction by

TABLE XXVI. *Maximal insulation* (I_0, *cm²sec°C/mcal*) *deduced from the basal metabolic rate and critical temperature according to equation 11, and expected insulation of the known layers of fat* (I_{fat}), *connective tissue* ($I_{conn.}$), *fur* (I_{fur}), *and free still air* (I_{air}), *summated to give an expected total insulation* (I_1)
Metabolic rates are taken from Table XXV, and critical temperatures from the authors quoted. The layer insulations are either taken from the measurements of these authors or deduced from the thickness of the layers, on the basis that $k_{fat} = 0.5$, $k_{conn.} = 0.9$, $k_{fur} = 0.09$, $k_{air} = 0.06$ mcal/cm sec°C.

Species	I_0	I_{fat}	$I_{conn.}$	I_{fur}	I_{air}	I_1	Reference
Densely furred							
Lemming	26	—	—	16	5	21	
Weasel	9	—	—	11	5	16	
Night monkey	14	—	—	19	5	24	Scholander *et al.*
Sloth	26	—	—	21	5	26	(1950a-c)
White fox	50	—	—	48	5	53	
Sheep (5 cm fleece)	19	—	—	55	5	60	Blaxter (1962)
Lightly furred							
Cow (0·8 cm hair)	13	—	6	9	5	20	Blaxter (1962)
Man	7	—	5	0	5	10	Gagge *et al.* (1938); Hertzmann (1961)
Pig	22	12	—	0	5	17	Irving (1956)
Aquatic							
Harbor seal	13	8	—	0	0	8	Irving and Hart (1957)

Dashes indicate where the insulation is unknown but believed to be small.

abandoning the countercurrent exchange system and stretching out its limbs, or it may evaporate water from its mouth. The former method is probably very effective for animals working hard in cold conditions, such as sled dogs or running caribou in the Arctic (Irving and Krog, 1954), but is of little use once the ambient air temperature rises to near that of the deep body, since then the temperature gradient is too small to allow much heat loss by conduction. Heat loss by evaporation starts at 20° C in the thickly fleeced sheep, and at 29–35° C in other species (Table XXV); the jerboa rat, with its long bare legs, is particularly well adapted to the use of conduction rather than evaporation for heat balance, and has the highest evaporation temperature. Oral evaporation takes two forms: dogs, cats and sheep pant (Hammel *et al.*, 1958; Prouty, 1949; Knapp and Robinson, 1954), while cats, rodents and at least one marsupial coat their fur with saliva (Prouty, 1949; Herrington, 1940; Kirmiz, 1962; Schmidt-Nielsen, 1954; Bartholomew, 1956). Saliva coating is relatively ineffective because much of the insulation of the animals is inside the surface from which evaporation takes place.

The densely furred animal has one advantage in heat stress: insulation affects it comparatively little, for the radiation is absorbed at the outer surface of the fur, and is mostly conducted and radiated out into the air again; under tropical sunlight the outer surface of a sheep's fleece can reach nearly 100° C (MacFarlane *et al.*, 1956).

HEAT BALANCE OF THINLY FURRED MAMMALS

This group includes all animals which have fur of insufficient density to keep out terrestrial winds. It includes many ungulates and monkeys. The three species which have been studied in detail are the domestic cow, pig and man.

The main insulation of a lightly furred mammal lies beneath the skin surface. This is illustrated by the critical temperature of the pig, which falls as its subcutaneous fat layer develops after birth (Table XXV). In the adult pig this fat layer accounts for most of the animal's insulation (Table XXVI). In the cow some of the insulation is in the fur (Table XXVI), but as the fur is not very dense it should be vulnerable to wind. Man has a thinner skin than these ungulates, so that he has remarkably little thermal insulation altogether (Table XXVI) and a correspondingly high critical temperature (Table XXV). Increase in subcutaneous fat increases his insulation and hence decreases his metabolic reaction to cold (Daniels and Baker, 1961). Because his subcutaneous insulation is poor, approximately half of a nude man's insulation lies in the free still air over his body, which is a very fragile barrier (Iampietro *et al.*, 1958). In primitive conditions man appears to adapt to cold stress mainly by raising his metabolic response and avoiding the exposure (Scholander *et al.*, 1958 a, b; Ward *et al.*, 1960; Elsner *et al.*, 1961). All three species allow their limbs to cool under cold stress, with countercurrent exchange of heat between the arteries and veins. In man this may result in loss of hand function, and adaptation consists of a forced heat loss by blood flow to the hand, rather than heat conservation (Elsner *et al.*, 1960, 1961). A high blood flow to the surface of the head is also maintained in the cold (Burton and Froese, 1957; Burton and Edwards, 1960b).

The absence of dense fur does not mean that an animal can exist without increased evaporation at a higher temperature; the evaporation temperature of the cow is only 24° C, and even in man evaporation starts at 33° C (Table XXV). The distinction lies in the type, and effectiveness, of the possible evaporation: evaporation is theoretically possible over the whole surface of of a thinly furred mammal. In practice, both its occurrence and distribution are variable. The pig appears unable to sweat in response to heat stress; it only pants (Mount, 1962, 1965). The cow sweats over the whole body, particularly on the shoulders (Taneja, 1959; Blaxter, 1962). Man sweats over the whole body to a pattern determined racially and individually (Kuno, 1956). Many other species sweat in heat stress but the distribution of their response is unknown. The evaporation of sweat over the whole body can produce an enormous heat loss. In man a loss of 15 mcal/cm^{2}sec can be maintained, which is 14 × the basal metabolism, and approximately equal to the maximum insolation possible, 14 mcal/cm^{2}sec if the fractional radiation area $\beta = 0.7$. Under optimum conditions human sweat evaporation is therefore capable of keeping heat balance even when the ambient temperature considerably exceeds that of the body (Adolph, 1947). The limit of a viable environment is only reached when the sweat cannot evaporate because the ambient vapour concentration approaches that at the skin surface (Eichna et al., 1945). In donkeys, camels and cows losses of 4–10 mcal/cm^{2}sec have been reported, also greatly in excess of their metabolic rates. In cows, this evaporation is supplemented by panting (Riek and Lee, 1948; Findlay, 1957).

In order to sustain this heat loss from the skin surface, the insulation of the skin must be greatly reduced; this is performed by the blood flow which cuts the insulation in man to less than 1 cm^{2}sec°C/mcal. Even this low insulation is sufficient to keep the skin surface relatively cool during maximal sweat evaporation.

The camel and rhinoceros allow their deep body temperature to rise by several degrees during a hot day, and thus conserve their body water at the expense of their heat balance (Schmidt-Nielsen et al., 1957; Allbrook et al., 1958). Man does not have this facility (Benzinger, 1959).

HEAT BALANCE OF AQUATIC MAMMALS

The insulation provided by water is negligible, so that with the exception of the fur seal and the diving rodents aquatic mammals are dependent on their subcutaneous fat for insulation. Although the fat is usually several cm thick it is not as good an insulator as fur, and provides only some one-fifth of the insulation of the Arctic mammals (Table XXVI). The low critical temperatures of seals in water (Table XXV) are mainly achieved by their abnormally high basal metabolic rate; the manatee, which has a low metabolic rate, is said to die in cool water despite its fat (Irving and Hart, 1957). The fur seal depends partially on its unwettable fur for insulation; juvenile seals, lacking this insulation, cannot live in cold water (Bartholomew and Wilke, 1956; Irving et al., 1962). Whales, being much larger, can afford a much thicker and therefore more effective layer of fat around their bodies. The insulation of the fat is not by-passed by the extremities, as can be seen by the greater value of I_0 than I_1 for the seal in Table XXVI. This is presumably due to the known countercurrent exchange system in the flippers, which is also present in the flukes and fins of whales.

Since evaporation cannot take place within water, aquatic mammals must rely on conduction to keep balance. Hair seals appear to operate their heat exchange in heat stress largely through the flippers (Irving and Hart, 1957), although the whole body surface is theoretically available for vascular convection. Fur seals, which find great difficulty in avoiding pyrexia on land (Irving et al., 1962), only inhabit water at <15° C; this may be a thermal limit. Seals on land lose heat by evaporation of sweat from their flippers (Bartholomew and Wilke, 1956).

Derivation of Membrane Capacity from Time Constant

CASE A

Assume a uniform membrane, thickness l, from $x = 0$ to $x = l$. At time $t = 0$, a solution of concentration C_0 is applied to the upper face of the membrane, and maintained at this concentration.

$$\text{i.e.} \qquad C = 0, \qquad x < 0$$

$$C = 0, \qquad t < 0$$

$$C = C_0, \qquad x = l, t \geqslant 0$$

Solving Fick's law, $\dfrac{\partial C}{\partial t} = D\dfrac{\partial^2 C}{\partial x^2}$, for these conditions, the concentration within the membrane will be:

$$C = \frac{C_0 x}{l} + \frac{2 C_0}{\pi} \sum_{n=1}^{\infty} (-1)^n \frac{1}{n} \sin\left(\frac{n\pi x}{l}\right) \exp\left(-\frac{n^2 \pi^2 Dt}{l^2}\right)$$

Crank (1956)

The first term is the equilibrium state, the second is the transient. A partition coefficient of unity is assumed.

Then

$$\frac{\partial C}{\partial x} = \frac{C_0}{l}\left(1 + 2 \sum_{n=1}^{\infty} (-1)^n \cos\frac{n\pi x}{l} \exp\left(-\frac{n^2 \pi^2 Dt}{l^2}\right)\right)$$

$\therefore$ the flow out of the membrane,

$$\frac{dq}{dt} = D\left(\frac{\partial C}{\partial x}\right)_{x=0}$$

$$= \frac{DC_0}{l}\left(1 + 2 \sum_{n=1}^{\infty} (-1)^n \exp\left(\frac{-n^2 \pi^2 Dt}{l^2}\right)\right)$$

145

And at time t

$$
\begin{aligned}
q &= \int_0^t D\left(\frac{\partial C}{\partial x}\right)_{x=0} dt \\
&= \frac{DC_0 t}{l} + 2DC_0 \sum_{n=1}^{\infty} (-1)^n \left[\frac{-l}{n^2\pi^2 D} \exp\left(\frac{-n^2\pi^2 Dt}{l^2}\right)\right]_0^t \\
&= \frac{DC_0 t}{l} - \frac{2lC_0}{\pi^2} \sum_{n=1}^{\infty} (-1)^n \frac{1}{n^2}\left(1 - \exp\left(\frac{-n^2\pi^2 Dt}{l^2}\right)\right)
\end{aligned}
$$

As t becomes large

$$
\begin{aligned}
q &\to \frac{DC_0 t - 2lC_0}{l} \frac{}{\pi^2}\left(1 - \frac{1}{4} + \frac{1}{9} - \cdots\right) \\
&= \frac{DC_0 t}{l} - \frac{lC_0}{6} \qquad \text{since } \sum_{n=1}^{\infty} (-1)^n \frac{1}{n^2} = \frac{\pi^2}{12}
\end{aligned}
$$

But

$$
\begin{aligned}
p &= \frac{1}{C_0}\left(\frac{dq}{dt}\right)_{t\to\infty} \\
&= \frac{D}{l}
\end{aligned}
$$

$$
\therefore \quad q \to pC_0 t - \frac{lC_0}{6}
$$

By definition of the delay period, t_d, at large times:

$$
q = pC_0(t - t_d)
$$

$$
\therefore \quad pt_d = \frac{l}{6}
$$

$$
l = 6pt_d \tag{1}
$$

If there is a partition between the solution and the membrane, such that the external concentration has to be αC_0 to maintain the above conditions, then

$$
\begin{aligned}
p &= \frac{1}{\alpha C_0}\left(\frac{dq}{dt}\right)_{t\to\infty} \\
&\doteqdot \frac{D}{\alpha l}
\end{aligned}
$$

$$
\therefore \quad l = 6\alpha pt_d \tag{1a}
$$

CASE B

(Originally described by Mr. M. Ainsworth)

Assume two thin membranes, each of thickness δ and permeability $2p$, separated by a well-stirred space of thickness l ($l \gg \delta$). The initial conditions are the same as in case **A**.

Let the concentration in the interval space be C_1

Then

$$l\frac{dC_1}{dt} = 2p(C_0 - 2C_1)$$

$\therefore$ For the given initial conditions

$$C_1 = \frac{C_0}{2}(1 - e^{-4pt/l})$$

$\therefore$ The quantity transferred through the lower membrane, q, is

$$q = 2p\int_0^t C_1\,dt$$

$$= pC_0\left(t - \frac{l}{4p}(1 - e^{-4pt/l})\right)$$

Again, by definition of t_d, at large times:

$$q = pC_0(t - t_d)$$

$$\therefore\ t_d = \frac{l}{4p}$$

$$l = 4\,pt_d \tag{2}$$

or again, if the interval-space is of a different solvent than the bulk solutions on each side of the thin membranes

$$l = 4\alpha\,pt_d \tag{2a}$$

Extension of a Diaphragm

A circular sheet of uniformly elastic tissue of radius a, thickness d, is held rigidly at its circumference. A pressure difference is applied across the diaphragm so formed, and the distension of the sheet is measured (Fig. 31C).

At the circumference, the tissue cannot stretch tangentially, so the peripheral extension must be entirely radial. At the centre extension is equal in all directions, by symmetry. It follows that the stretch of the diaphragm is non-uniform. In order to handle this system mathematically, it is necessary to neglect this non-uniformity, and to assume that the region of restricted extension is small relative to that of free extension.

In this case, the radius of curvature b of the tissue over the entire diaphragm would be constant, again by symmetry. By a classical proof the static stress T within a shell due to its curvature under a pressure difference is:

$$T = \frac{pb}{2d} \qquad \text{(1: Champion and Davy, 1952)}$$

The strain (S) in the tissue is

$$S = \frac{l-a}{a} \qquad (2)$$

where $2l$ = length across the distended sheet (Fig. 31D; p. 74).

Now
$$\frac{l}{b} = \sin^{-1}\frac{a}{b}$$

$$= \frac{a}{b}\left(1+\frac{a^2}{6b^2}+ \cdots \right)$$

Neglecting powers a in $\frac{a^4}{b^4}$ and above

$$l \doteqdot a\left(1+\frac{a^2}{6b^2}\right)$$

Substituting in equation 2

$$S \doteqdot \frac{a^2}{6b^2} \tag{3}$$

Again, by geometry (Fig. 31D):

$$b = \frac{x^2 + a^2}{2x}$$

where x is the displacement of the centre of the sheet.
Substituting for b in equations 1 and 3

$$T = \frac{pa^2}{4xd}\left(1 + \frac{x^2}{a^2}\right) \tag{4}$$

$$S \doteqdot \frac{2x^2}{3a^2(1 + x^2/a^2)^2}$$

Neglecting the term in x^4/a^4,

$$S \doteqdot \frac{2x^2}{3a^2(1 + 2x^2/a^2)} \tag{5}$$

Slip of Rods in a Viscous Liquid

A set of uniform rods, length x and radius r, are arranged parallel to one another in a regular rectangular array within a Newtonian liquid of viscosity η. Each rod overlaps its neighbours by half its length, so that the whole array consists of n sets, each staggered by half its length from the neighbouring sets (Fig. 42; p. 91). The total length of the system is:

$$l = \frac{x}{2}(n+1) \tag{1}$$

Let the space between the centres of adjacent rods be h. The number of rods of a given set per unit cross-sectional area is then

$$m = \frac{1}{2h^2} \tag{2}$$

Each rod is surrounded by four others of the adjacent set (Fig. 42B).

The nth set of rods is pulled away from the system by a stress T; at dynamic equilibrium it reaches a velocity v. Each set of rods slides relative to the adjacent sets with a velocity Δv, such that

$$\Delta v = \frac{v}{n-1} \tag{3}$$

If $n \gg 1$, substituting from (1) into (3)

$$\Delta v \fallingdotseq \frac{vx}{2l} \tag{4}$$

It is not possible to calculate the fluid friction between each rod and its four neighbours simply, since the geometry of the velocity profile is complicated. Since the system is Newtonian, the force (q) must be given approximately by:

$$q = \frac{2\pi r x \eta \Delta v}{f(h,r)}$$

Where $f(h, r)$ is the "effective distance" between the moving surfaces.

150

The force on the entire set of m rods is equal to the stress, since the system is in steady motion

$$\therefore \quad T = \frac{2 m \pi \eta \, xr \, \Delta v}{f}$$

Substituting for m from equation (2) and for Δv from equation (4)

$$T = \frac{\pi \eta \, x^2 \, rv}{2 h^2 f l}$$

$$\therefore \quad \frac{v}{lT} = \frac{2 h^2 f}{\pi \eta \, x^2 \, r} \tag{5}$$

$$= u, \text{ the viscous extensibility}$$

If one assumes that the effective spacing is twice the minimum distance between the rods

$$f = 2(h - 2r)$$

$$\frac{v}{lT} = \frac{4 h^2 (h - 2r)}{\pi \eta \, x^2 \, r} \tag{6}$$

N.B. The assumed dynamic equilibrium only lasts so long as the absolute movement of the rods is too small to affect their overlap significantly.

Viscous Flow between a Set of Stacks of Parallel Plates

The flow of a Newtonian liquid from between two parallel circular plates of radius a, separated by a distance x and pressed together by a force P for a time t is given by

$$\left(\frac{x_0}{x}\right)^2 = 1 + \frac{4Px_0{}^2 t}{3\pi\eta a^4}$$

(Reynolds, 1886, quoted by Barr, 1931). For a stack of such plates of total height h

$$\left(\frac{h_0}{h}\right)^2 = 1 + \frac{4Px_0{}^2 t}{3\pi\eta a^4}$$

Suppose n such stacks are rectangularly close-packed within a circle of radius r (Fig. 43; p. 93). Then if $r \gg a$

$$r^2 \doteqdot \frac{4n}{\pi} a^2$$

The force on each stack is $\quad F/n = \dfrac{4a^2 F}{\pi r^2}$

$$\therefore \quad \left(\frac{h_0}{h}\right)^2 = 1 + \frac{16 F x_0{}^2 t}{3\pi^2 \eta r^2 a^2} \tag{1}$$

When $\qquad h = \dfrac{h_0}{2},\ t = t_{\frac{1}{2}};$

$$t_{\frac{1}{2}} = \frac{9\pi^2 \eta r^2 a^2}{16 F x_0{}^2} \tag{2}$$

N.B. In this system it has been assumed that viscous resistance to fluid outside the stacks, in its further progress to the periphery r, is negligible.

Incident and Absorbed Energy

In a homogeneous medium the radiation transmitted is given by the relation:

$$I(x) = I_0 e^{-x/\lambda} \tag{1}$$

where I_0 = incident energy

$I(x)$ = energy incident at depth x.

The energy absorbed per unit mass of the medium is given by:

$$Q(x) = -\frac{1}{\rho}\frac{dI}{dx} \qquad (\rho = \text{density})$$

$$= \frac{I_0}{\lambda\rho} e^{-x/\lambda}$$

∴ Near the surface of the medium

$$Q_0 = \frac{I_0}{\lambda\rho} \tag{2}$$

For skin $\rho \doteqdot 1\cdot2$ g/ml (Vennart, 1954)

$$\therefore \quad Q_0 = 0\cdot8\ I_0/\lambda \tag{3}$$

For X-rays of energy 100 keV, $\lambda \doteqdot 6$ cm (Grodstein, 1957) so that
1 rad (100 keV) $\equiv 18\ \mu\text{cal/cm}^2$

Countercurrent Heat Exchange

Consider a tissue layer, thickness l, containing a countercurrent flow system through which passes a mass flow m per unit cross-sectional area of the tissue (Fig. 62).

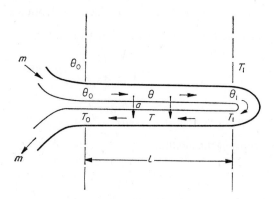

FIG. 62. Idealized countercurrent thermal exchange system between an artery and vein.

Let the temperature difference across the tissue layer be $\theta_0 - T_1$, and the conductance across the exchange system be a per unit length of tube.

Then, since the heat lost by the outgoing fluid equals that gained by the ingoing fluid

$$\theta_0 - \theta_1 = T_0 - T_1 \quad (cf. \text{ Fig. 62})$$

$$\therefore \quad \theta_0 - T_0 = \theta_1 - T_1$$

$$= \theta - T$$

i.e. there is a constant temperature difference between the tubes throughout the system.

The heat flow from one tube to the other (H_1) is

$$H_1 = al\,(\theta - T)$$

154

The heat flow across the tissue layer due to the mass flow (H_2) is

$$H_2 = ms(\theta - T) \quad (s = \text{specific heat of fluid})$$
$$= ms(\theta_0 - T_1) - H_1$$
$$= ms(\theta_0 - T_1) - al(\theta - T)$$

$$\therefore \quad \frac{ms}{al + ms} = \frac{\theta - T}{\theta_0 - T_1} \tag{1}$$

Now the effective conductance of the mass flow (C_m) is given by:

$$C_m = \frac{H_2}{\theta_0 - T_1}$$

$$= \frac{ms(\theta - T)}{\theta_0 - T_1}$$

$$= ms \cdot \frac{ms}{al + ms} \qquad \text{from equation 1}$$

$$= \frac{ms}{1 + \alpha} \tag{2}$$

$$\text{where} \quad \alpha = \frac{al}{ms}$$

Thermal Exchange by Radiation between a Black Body and its Radiant Environment

A black body at an absolute temperature T emits energy at a rate M per unit area, where:

$$M = \sigma T^4$$

The radiant exchange between two such bodies whose temperatures differ by ΔT, and which radiate completely to one another, is given by:

$$M = H_R$$
$$= \sigma((T+\Delta T)^4 - T^4)$$

If ΔT is small relative to T, then

$$H_R = 4\sigma T^3 \cdot \Delta T$$

$$\therefore \quad \frac{H_R}{\Delta T} = C_R, \text{ the radiative conductance}$$

$$= 4\sigma T^3$$

Now $\sigma = 5\cdot70 \times 10^{-12}$ watts. cm². °K^{-4} (Roberts and Miller, 1951)

$$\therefore \text{ at } T = 305°\,K\ (32°\,C),$$
$$C_R = 0\cdot154 \text{ mcal/cm}^2\text{sec°C}$$
$$\text{and at } T = 295°\,K\ (22°\,C)$$
$$C_R = 0\cdot140 \text{ mcal/cm}^2\text{sec°C}$$

References

Adams, P. D. (1949). The gas exchange of the skin. *Am. Perfumer ess. Oil Rev.*, pp. 134–137.

Adolph, E. A. (1947). "Physiology of Man in the Desert." Interscience, New York.

Ainsworth, M. (1960). Methods for measuring percutaneous absorption. *J. Soc. cosmet. Chem.* **11**, 69–78.

Albert, R. E. and Palmes, E. D. (1951). Evaporative rate patterns from small skin areas as measured by an infra-red gas analyser. *J. appl. Physiol.* **4**, 208–214.

Alexander, G. and Williams, D. (1962). Heat exchange in lambs in a hot environment. *Aust. J. agric. Res.* **13**, 122–143.

Alexander, P. and Earland, C. (1950). The sub-cuticle membrane; a recently discovered morphological component of the wool fibre. *Text. Res. J.* **20**, 298–300.

Allbrook, D. B., Harthoorn, A. M., Luck, C. P. and Wright, P. G. (1958). Temperature regulation in the white rhinoceros. *J. Physiol.* **143**, 51–52P.

Aman, A. (1962). Accidental poisoning from agricultural pesticides. *Bull. Wld Hlth Org.* **26**, 109–120.

Aoki, T. (1955). Stimulation of the sweat glands in the hairy skin of the dog by adrenaline, noradrenaline, acetylcholine, mecholyl and pilocarpine. *J. invest. Dermat.* **24**, 545–556.

Aschoff, J. and Kaempffer, F. (1947). Wärmedurchgang durch die Haut und seine Änderung bei Vasokonstriktion. *Pflügers Arch. ges. Physiol.* **249**, 112–124.

Aschoff, J. and Wever, R. (1959). Anisotropy of the skin's conductivity. *Pflügers Arch. ges. Physiol.* **269**, 130–134.

Axelrod, D. J. and Hamilton, J. G. (1947). Radio-autographic studies of the distribution of lewisite and mustard gas in skin and eye tissues. *Am. J. Path.* **23**, 389–411.

Bachem, H. and Reed, C. I. (1931). The penetration of light through human skin. *Am. J. Physiol.* **97**, 86–91.

Baden, H. P. and Pearlman, C. (1964). The effect of ultra-violet light on protein and nucleic acid synthesis in the epidermis. *J. invest. Derm.* **43**, 71–75.

Banfield, W. G. and Brindley, D. C. (1963). Preliminary observations on senile elastosis using the electron microscope. *J. invest. Derm.* **41**, 9–17.

Barnett, A. (1938). The phase angle of normal human skin. *J. Physiol.* **93**, 349–366.

Barnett, C. H., Harrison, R. J. and Tomlinson, J. D. W. (1958). Variations in the venous systems of mammals. *Biol. Rev.* **33**, 442–487.

Barr, G. (1931). "A Monograph of Viscometry." Oxford University Press, London.

Barrer, R. M. (1951). "Diffusion in and through Solids." Cambridge University Press, London.

Barrnett, R. J. (1962). Morphology of adipose tissue with particular reference to its histochemistry and ultrastructure. *In* "Adipose Tissue as an Organ" (L. W. Kinsell, ed.), pp. 3–78. Thomas, Springfield.

Barron, E. S. G., Meyer, J. and Baker Miller, Z. (1948). The metabolism of the skin; effect of vesicant agents. *J. invest. Derm.* **11,** 97–118.

Bartholomew, G. A. (1956). Temperature regulation in the macropod marsupial *Setonix brachyurus. Physiol. Zoöl.* **29,** 26–40.

Bartholomew, G. A. and Wilke, F. (1956). Body temperature in the fur seal. *J. Mammal.* **37,** 327–337.

Baumberger, J. P., Suntzeff, V. and Cowdry, E. V. (1941). Methods for the separation of epidermis from dermis and some physiological and chemical properties of isolated epidermis. *J. natn. Cancer Inst.* **11,** 413–423.

Bazett, H. C., Love, L., Newton, M., Eisenberg, L., Day, R. and Forster, R. (1949). Temperature changes in blood flowing in arteries and veins in man. *J. appl. Physiol.* **1,** 3–19.

Beament, J. W. L. (1961a). Electrical properties of orientated lipid as a biological membrane. *Nature, Lond.* **191,** 217–221.

Beament, J. W. L. (1961b). The water relations of insect cuticle. *Biol. Rev.* **36,** 281–320.

Bearman, R. J. (1961). On the molecular basis of some current theories of diffusion. *J. phys. Chem.* **65,** 1961–1968.

Bennett, J. W. and Hutchinson, J. C. D. (1964). Thermal insulation of short lengths of merino fleeces. *Aust. J. agric. Res.* **15,** 427–445.

Bensley, S. H. (1934). On the presence, properties and distribution of the inter-cellular ground substance of loose connective tissue. *Anat. Rec.* **60,** 93.

Benzinger, T. H. (1959). Physical heat regulation and the sense of temperature in man. *Proc. natn. Acad. Sci. U.S.A.* **45,** 645–659.

Benzinger, T. H. and Kitzinger, C. (1949). Direct calorimetry by means of the gradient principle. *Rev. scient. Instrum.* **20,** 849–860.

Berenson, G. S. and Burch, G. E. (1951). Studies of diffusion of water through dead human skin. *Am. J. trop. Med.* **31,** 842–853.

Bernhardt, E. C. (1959). "Processing of Thermoplastic Materials", pp. 500–501. Reinhold, New York.

Bettley, F. R. (1961). The influence of soap on the permeability of the epidermis. *Br. J. Derm.* **73,** 448–454.

Bettley, F. R. (1963). The irritant effect of soap in relation to epidermal permeability. *Br. J. Derm.* **75,** 113–116.

Bettley, F. R. and Donoghue, E. (1960). Effect of soap on the diffusion of water through isolated human epidermis. *Nature, Lond.* **185,** 17–20.

Bidstrup, P. L. and Payne, D. J. H. (1951). Poisoning by di-nitro-ortho-cresol. *Br. med. J.* **1,** 16–19.

Biedermann, W. (1928). Protective and structural integument of lower vertebrates and the plumage of birds. *Ergebn. Biol.* **3,** 354–541.

Birbeck, M. S. C., Breathnack, A. S. and Everall, J. D. (1961). An electron microscope study of basal melanocytes and high-level clear cells in vitiligo. *J. invest. Derm.* **37,** 51–64.

Blank, H., Smith, J. G. and Fischer, R. W. (1961). The epidermal barrier: a comparison between scrotal and abdominal skin. *J. invest. Derm.* **36,** 337–341.

Blank, I. H. (1939). Measurement of pH of the skin surface. *J. invest. Derm.* **2,** 67–79.

Blank, I. H. (1952). Factors which influence the water content of the stratum corneum. *J. invest. Derm.* **18,** 433–440.

Blank, I. H. (1953). Further observations on factors which influence the water content of the stratum corneum. *J. invest. Derm.* **21**, 259–269.

Blank, I. H. and Finesinger, J. E. (1946). Electrical resistance of the skin. *Archs Neurol. Psychiat.* **56**, 544–557.

Blank, I. H. and Gould, E. (1959). Penetration of sodium laurate and sodium dodecyl sulphate into excised human skin. *J. invest. Derm.* **33**, 327–336.

Blank, I. H. and Gould, E. (1962). Study of mechanisms which impede the penetration of synthetic anionic surfactants into skin. *J. invest. Derm.* **37**, 311–315.

Blank, I. H. and Scheuplein, R. J. (1964). The epidermal barrier. *In* "Progress in the Biological Sciences in Relation to Dermatology", 2nd ed. (A. J. Rook and R. H. Champion, eds.), Vol. 2. Cambridge University Press, London.

Blank, I. H. and Shappiro, E. B. (1955). Effect of previous contact with aqueous solutions of soaps and detergents on the water content of the stratum corneum. *J. invest. Derm.* **25**, 391–401.

Blank, I. H., Griesemer, R. D. and Gould, E. (1957). The penetration of sarin into excised human skin. *J. invest. Derm.* **29**, 299–309.

Blank, I. H., Griesemer, R. D. and Gould, E. (1958a). Autoradiographic studies on the penetration of sarin into skin. *J. invest. Derm.* **30**, 187–191.

Blank, I. H., Griesemer, R. D. and Gould, E. (1958b). A method for studying the rate of sarin penetration into the living rabbit. *J. invest. Derm.* **31**, 255–258.

Blank, I. H., Jones, J. L. and Gould, E. (1958c). A study of the penetration of aluminium salts into excised human skin. *Proc. Toilet Goods Ass.* **29**.

Blank, I. H., Gould, E. and Theobald, A. (1964). Penetration of cationic surfactants into skin. *J. invest. Derm.* **42**, 363–366.

Blaxter, K. L. (1962). "The Energy Metabolism of Ruminants." Hutchinson, London.

Blaxter, K. L., Graham, N. McC. and Wainman, F. W. (1959). The metabolism and thermal exchanges of sheep with fleeces. *J. agric. Sci., Camb.* **52**, 41–49.

Blix, G. and Snellman, O. (1947). On chondroitin sulphuric acid and hyaluronic acid. *Chem. Abstr.* **41**, 1260.

Blum, H. F. and Terus, W. S. (1946). The erythemal threshold for sunburn. *Am. J. Physiol.* **146**, 107–117.

Blum, H. F., Watrous, W. G. and West, R. J. (1935). On the mechanism of photo-sensitization in man. *Am. J. Physiol.* **113**, 350–353.

Blum, H. F., Baer, R. L. and Sulzberger, M. B. (1946). Studies in hypersensitivity to light. *J. invest. Derm.* **7**, 99–108.

Born, W. C. (1958). Beseitigung radioaktiver vernunreinigungen in der Haut des Menschen. *Strahlentherapie* **106**, 435–445.

Borysko, E. (1963). Collagen. *In* "Ultrastructure of Protein Fibres" (R. Borasky, ed.), pp. 19–34. Academic Press, New York.

Bowes, J. H. and Kenten, R. H. (1949). The amino-acid distribution of collagen, elastin and reticular tissue. *Biochem. J.* **43**, 358–365.

Braun-Falco, O. and Rupec, M. (1964). Some observations on dermal collagen fibrils in ultra-thin sections. *J. invest. Derm.* **42**, 15–19.

Breathnack, A. S. (1964). The dermo-epidermal junction. *In* "Progress in the Biological Sciences in Relation to Dermatology", 2nd ed. (A. Rook and R. H. Champion, eds.), Cambridge University Press, London.

Breuer, H. (1924). Über die Wärmeleitung des Muskels und Fettes. *Pflüg. Arch. ges. Physiol.* **204**, 442–447.

Brinkman, R. and Lambert, H. B. (1958). Direct registration of an instantaneous X-ray effect in rats and man. *Nature, Lond.* **181**, 774–775.

Brody, I. (1959). The keratinization of epidermal cells of normal guinea-pig skin as revealed by electron microscopy. *J. Ultrastruct. Res.* **2**, 482–511.

Brody, I. (1960). The ultrastructure of the tonofibrils in the keratinization process of normal human epidermis. *J. Ultrastruct. Res.* **4**, 264–297.

Brody, I. (1962). The ultrastructure of the epidermis in psoriasis vulgaris. *J. Ultrastruct. Res.* **6**, 304–367.

Brook, A. H. and Short, B. F. (1960). Sweating in sheep. *Aust. J. agric. Res.* **11**, 557–569.

Brück, K. and Hensel, H. (1953). Heat flow and internal temperature in human limbs. *Pflüg. Arch. ges. Physiol.* **257**, 70–86.

Buck, H. W., Magnus, I. A. and Porter, A. D. (1960). The action spectrum of 8-methoxy psoralen for erythema in human skin. *Br. J. Derm.* **72**, 249–255.

Buettner, K. J. K. (1951). Effects of extreme heat and cold on human skin. *J. appl. Physiol.* **3**, 691–713.

Buettner, K. J. K. (1953). Diffusion of water and water vapour through human skin. *J. appl. Physiol.* **6**, 229–242.

Buettner, K. J. K. (1959a). Diffusion of liquid water through human skin. *J. appl. Physiol.* **14**, 261–268.

Buettner, K. J. K. (1959b). Diffusion of water vapour through small areas of human skin in a normal environment. *J. appl. Physiol.* **14**, 269–275.

Bull, H. B. (1957). Protein structure and elasticity. *In* "Tissue Elasticity" (J. Remington, ed.), pp. 33–43. American Physiological Society Publication.

Burch, G. E. and de Pasquale, N. P. (1962). "Hot Climates, Man and his Heart." Thomas, Springfield.

Burch, G. E. and Sodemann, W. A. (1944). Regional variations in water loss from skin of diseased subjects living in a subtropical climate. *J. clin. Invest.* **23**, 37–43.

Burch, G. E. and Winsor, T. (1944). Diffusion of water through dead plantar, palmar and dorsal human skin and through the toe nails. *Archs Derm. Syph.* **53**, 39–41.

Burch, G. E. and Winsor, T. (1946). Rate of insensible perspiration locally through living and dead human skin. *Archs intern. Med.* **74**, 437–444.

Burgess, G. H. (1956). The absence of keratin in teleost epithelium. *Nature, Lond.* **178**, 93–94.

Burns, R. C. (1950). A study of skin impedance. *Electronics*, pp. 190–196.

Burton, A. C. (1954). Relation of structure to function of the tissue of the walls of blood vessels. *Physiol. Rev.* **34**, 619–642.

Burton, A. C. and Edholm, O. G. (1955). "Man in a Cold Environment." Arnold, London.

Burton, A. C. and Edwards, M. (1960a). Correlation of heat output and blood flow in the finger. *J. appl. Physiol.* **15**, 201–208.

Burton, A. C. and Edwards, M. (1960b). Temperature distribution over the human head. *J. appl. Physiol.* **15**, 209–211.

Burton, A. C. and Froese, G. (1957). Heat losses from the human head. *J. appl. Physiol.* **10**, 235–241.

Butcher, E. O. and Cronin, A. (1949). The physical properties of human sebum. *J. invest. Derm.* **12**, 249–254.

Butterfield, W. J., Drake Seager, E. R., Dixey, J. R. and Treadwell, E. E. (1956). Observations on flash burning of human subjects in the laboratory using infrared and predominantly white light sources. *Surg. Gynec. Obstet.* **103**, 655–665.

Calvery, H. O., Deraize, J. H. and Laug, E. P. (1946). The metabolism and permeability of normal skin. *Physiol. Rev.* **26**, 495–540.

Carter, H. B. and Clarke, W. H. (1957). The hair follicle group and skin follicle population of sheep. *Aust. J. agric. Res.* **8**, 91–119.

Causey, G. (1962). "Electron Microscopy." Livingstone, Edinburgh.

Chalmers, T. M. (1964). Structure and metabolism of adipose tissue. *In* "Progress in the Biological Sciences in Relation to Dermatology" (A. Rook and R. H. Champion, eds.), pp. 165–174. Cambridge University Press, London.

Champion, F. C. and Davy, N. (1952). "Properties of Matter." Blackie, London.

Charles, A. (1959). An electron microscope study of cornification in the human skin. *J. invest. Derm.* **33**, 65–74.

Charles, A. and Smiddy, F. G. (1957). Tonofibrils of the human epidermis. *J. invest. Derm.* **29**, 327–338.

Choman, B. R. (1960). Autoradiographic studies on percutaneous absorption. *J. Soc. cosmet. Chem.* **11**, 127–137.

Ciferri, A., Puett, D. and Rajagh, L. V. (1965). Elasticity of collagen tendons. *Biopolymers* **3**, 439–459.

Clark, C., Vinegar, R. and Hardy, J. D. (1953). Goniometric spectrometer for the measurement of diffuse reflectance and transmittance of skin in the infra-red spectral region. *J. opt. Soc. Am.* **43**, 993–998.

Clark, J. H. (1936). The temperature coefficient of the production of erythema by ultra-violet radiation. *Am. J. Hyg.* **113**, 334–342.

Cleves, A. C. and Sumner, J. F. (1962). The measurement of human capacitance and resistance in relation to electrostatic hazards with primary explosives. *Explos. Res. Dev. Establ. Rep.* 18 R.62.

Coblentz, W. W., Stair, R. and Hogue, J. M. (1932). The spectral reaction of the untanned human skin to ultra-violet radiation. *U.S. Bur. Stand. J. Res.* **8**, 541–547.

Cohen, M. (1961). Depth-dose tables for use in radiotherapy. *Br. J. Radiol.* Suppl. 10.

Cole, K. S. (1932). Electric phase angle of cell membranes. *J. gen. Physiol.* **15**, 641–649.

Conn, J. W. (1949). The mechanism of acclimatization to heat. *Adv. intern. Med.* **3**, 373–393.

Cotty, V. F., Skerpac, J., Ederma, H. M., Zurzola, F. and Kuna, M. (1960). The percutaneous absorption of salicylates as measured by blood plasma levels in the rabbit. *J. Soc. cosmet. Chem.* **11**, 97–116.

Coulson, C. A. (1952). "Valence", pp. 186 and 308. Oxford University Press, London.

Cragg, J. B. and Davies, L. (1947). Sweating in sheep. *Nature, Lond.* **159**, 34–35.

Craig, F. N. (1956). Uptake or output of water by the skin as influenced by external vapour pressure in liquid or vapour contact and by atropine. *J. appl. Physiol.* **8**, 473–477.

Crank, J. (1955). Some methods of deducing the diffusion coefficient and its concentration dependence from sorption experiments. *Trans. Faraday Soc.* **51**, 1632–1641.

Crank, J. (1956). "The Mathematics of Diffusion." Oxford University Press, London.

Crank, J. and Park, G. S. (1949). An evaluation of the diffusion coefficient for chloroform in polystyrene from simple absorption experiments. *Trans. Faraday Soc.* **45**, 240–249.

Crew, W. H. and Whittle, C. H. (1938). On the absorption of ultra-violet radiation by human sweat. *J. Physiol.* **93**, 335–348.

Cruikshank, C. N. D. and Hell, E. A. (1963). The effect of injury upon the uptake of tritiated thymidine by guinea pig epidermis. *Expl. Cell Res.* **31**, 128–139.

Daniels, F. (1959). The physiological effects of sunlight. *J. invest. Derm.* **32**, 147–155.

Daniels, F. and Baker, P. T. (1961). Relationship between body fat and shivering in air at 15° C. *J. appl. Physiol.* **16**, 421–425.

Daniels, F., Drophy, D. and Lobitz, W. C. (1961). Histochemical response of human skin following ultra-violet irradiation. *J. invest. Derm.* **37**, 351–357.

Darrow, C. W. (1929). The galvanic skin reflex and skin volume changes. *Am. J. Physiol.* **88**, 219–229.

Davson, H. and Danielli, J. F. (1952). "The Permeability of Natural Membranes", 2nd ed. Cambridge University Press, London.

Day, T. D. (1949). The mode of reaction of interstitial connective tissue with water. *J. Physiol.* **109**, 380–391.

Day, T. D. (1952). The effect of hyaluronidase on the flow of water in connective tissue. *In* "Deformation and Flow in Biological Systems" (A. Frey-Wyssling, ed.), pp. 503–505. North-Holland Publishing Co., Amsterdam.

Dempsey, M. (1946). Sweat glands. *Nature, Lond.* **157**, 5B.

De Long, C. W., Thompson, R. C. and Kornberg, H. A. (1954). Percutaneous absorption of tritium oxide. *Am. J. Roentg.* **71**, 1038–1045.

Dick, J. C. (1951). Stretch-resistance of skin. *J. Physiol.* **112**, 102–113.

Dickerson, R. E. (1964). X-ray analysis and protein structure. *In* "The Proteins" (H. Neurath and K. Bailey, eds.), Vol. 2, p. 746. Academic Press, New York and London.

Dimitroff, J. M., Kuppenheim, H. F., Graham, I. C. and McKeehan, C. W. (1955). Spectral reflectance of the skin of rats, rabbits and hairless mice in the regions 243–700 mμ and 0·707–2·66 μ. *J. appl. Physiol.* **8**, 532–534.

Dirnhuber, P. and Tregear, R. T. (1960). Equilibration between water vapour and human skin. *J. Physiol.* **152**, 58–59P.

Dobson, R. L. and Bosley, L. (1963). The effect of keratinase on human epidermis. *J. invest. Derm.* **41**, 131–134.

Dodson, J. W. (1963). On the nature of tissue interactions in embryonic skin. *Expl. Cell Res.* **31**, 233–235.

Dowling, D. F. (1956). Hair follicle density in cattle. *Aust. J. agric. Res.* **6**, 645–654.

Draize, J. H. (1942). The determination of the pH of the skin of man and common laboratory animals. *J. invest. Derm.* **5**, 77–85.

Draize, J. H. and Kelley, E. A. (1959). Urinary excretion of boric acid preparations following oral and topical administration to rabbits. *Toxicol. appl. Pharmac.* **1**, 267–276.

Dry, F. W. (1925). The coat of the mouse. *J. Genet.* **16**, 287–340.

Dry, F. W. (1928). Agouti mice and rats. *J. Genet.* **20**, 131–144.

DuBois, D. and Dubois, E. F. (1915). The measurement of the surface area of man. *Archs intern. Med.* **15**, 868–881.

Durham, W. F. and Wolffe, H. R. (1962). Measurement of the exposure of workers to pesticides. *Bull. Wld Hlth Org.* **26**, 75–91.

Durham, W. F., Wolffe, H. R., Walker, K. C. and Elliott, J. W. (1959). Evaluation of the health hazards involved in house spraying with DDT. *Bull. Wld Hlth Org.* **20**, 1–14.

Ebbecke, U. (1921). The local galvanic reaction of the skin. *Arch. Physiol.* **190**, 230–269.

Ebling, F. J. (1964). The hair follicle. *In* "Progress in the Biological Sciences in Relation to Dermatology", 2nd ed. (A. Rook and R. H. Champion, eds.), pp. 303–324. Cambridge University Press, London.

Edelberg, R. (1964). The contribution of the epidermis to the exosomatic GSR as determined by microelectrodes. (Unpublished observations.)

Edelberg, R., Greiner, T. and Burch, N. R. (1960). Some membrane properties in the galvanic skin response. *Archs Neurol. Psychiat.* **7**, 163–169.

Edwards, E. A. and Duntley, S. A. (1939). The pigments and colour of living human skin. *Am. J. Anat.* **65**, 1–34.

Edwards, E. A., Finkelstein, N. A. and Duntley, S. Q. (1951). Spectrophotometry of living human skin. *J. invest. Derm.* **16**, 311–321.

Eichna, L. W., Ashe, W. F., Bean, W. B. and Shelley, W. B. (1945). Upper limits of environmental heat tolerance. *J. ind. Hyg. Toxicol.* **27**, 59–84.

Einbinder, J. M. and Walzer, R. A. (1963). Separation of epidermis from dermis by use of disodium cantharides. *J. invest. Derm.* **41**, 109.

Ellis, R. A. (1961). Vascular patterns of the skin. *Adv. Biol. Skin* **2**, 20–37.

Elod, E. and Zahn, H. (1946). Die Loslichkeit chemisch behandelter Schafwolle in Pankreatin. *Melliands Textber.* **27**, 68–70.

Elsner, R. W., Nelms, J. D. and Irving, L. (1960). Circulation of heat to the hands of Arctic Indians. *J. appl. Physiol.* **15**, 662–666.

Elsner, R. W., Milan, F. A. and Rodahl, K. (1961). Thermal and metabolic responses of men in the Antarctic to a standard cold stress. *J. appl. Physiol.* **16**, 401–404.

Enger, P. S. (1957). Heat regulation and metabolism in some tropical mammals and birds. *Acta physiol. scand.* **40**, 161–166.

Evans, T. C., Goodrich, J. P. and Slaughter J. C. (1942). Temperature and radio-sensitivity of skin of new-born rats. *Radiology* **38**, 201–206.

Evans, E. I., Brooks, J. W., Schmidt, F. H., Williams, R. C. and Ham, W. T. (1955). Flash burn studies on human volunteers. *Surgery* **37**, 280–297.

Faires, R. A. and Parkes, B. H. (1960). "Radioisotope Laboratory Techniques." Newnes, London.

Fawcett, D. W. (1942). A comparative study of blood vascular bundles in the Florida manatee and in certain cetaceans and edentates. *J. Morph.* **71**, 105–124.

Felsher, Z. (1947). Studies on the adherence of the epidermis to the corneum. *J. Invest. Derm.* **8**, 35–47.

Ferguson, K. A. and Dowling, D. F. (1956). The function of cattle sweat glands. *Aust. J. agric. Res.* **6**, 640–644.

Fessler, J. H. (1960). A structural function of mucopolysaccharides in connective tissue. *Biochem. J.* **76**, 124–131.

Finck, J. L. (1930). Mechanism of heat flow in fibrous materials. *Bur. Stand. J. Res.* **5**, 973–984.

Findlay, J. D. (1957). The respiratory activity of calves subjected to thermal stress. *J. Physiol.* **136**, 300–309.

Findlay, J. D. and Jenkinson, D. McE. (1960). The sweat glands of the bovine. *J. agric. Sci.* **55**, 247–249.

Fine, S., Klein, E., Farber, S., Scott, R. E., Roy, A. and Seed, R. E. (1963). *In vivo* effects of laser radiation on the skin of the golden hamster. *J. invest. Derm.* **40**, 123–124.

Fitton-Jackson, S. (1953). Fibrogenesis *in vivo* and *in vitro*. *In* "Nature and Structure of Collagen" (J. T. Randall, ed.), pp. 140–151. Butterworth, London.

Fitzgerald, L. R. (1957). Cutaneous respiration. *Physiol. Rev.* **37**, 325–336.

Flesch, P. (1958). Chemical data on human epidermal keratinization and differentiation. *J. invest. Derm.* **31**, 63–73.

Flesch, P. (1963). Inhibition of keratinizing structures by systemic drugs. *Pharmac. Rev.* **15**, 653–671.

Flesch, P. and Esoda, E. C. J. (1960). Mucopolysaccharides in human epidermis. *J. invest. Derm.* **35**, 43–46.

Flesch, P. and Esoda, E. C. J. (1962). Isolation of a glycoproteolipid from human horny layers. *J. invest. Derm.* **39**, 409–415.

Flesch, P. and Roe, D. A. (1960). The Gram-staining material of human epidermis. *J. invest. Derm.* **34**, 17–28.

Fletcher, T. E., Press, J. M. and Wilson, D. B. (1959). Exposure of spraymen to dieldrin in residual spraying. *Bull. Wld Hlth Org.* **20**, 15–25.

Folk, G. E. and Peary, R. E. (1951). Water penetration into the foot. Quartermaster Climatic Research Laboratory Report, No. 181.

Forster, R. E., Ferris, B. G. and Day, R. (1946). Heat exchange and blood flow in the hand. *Am. J. Physiol.* **146**, 600–609.

Fox, R. H., Goldsmith, R., Hampton, I. F. G. and Lewis, H. E. (1964). The nature of the increase in sweating capacity produced by acclimatization. *J. Physiol.* **171**, 368–376.

Fredriksonn, T. (1958). Studies on the percutaneous absorption of sarin and two allied organophosphorous cholinesterase inhibitors. *Acta derm.-vener.* **38**, Suppl. 41.

Fredriksonn, T. (1962a). The rate of percutaneous absorption of paraoxon. *J. invest. Derm.* **38**, 233–236.

Fredriksonn, T. (1962b). The rate of percutaneous absorption of parathion. *Acta derm.-vener.* **41**, 353–362.

Freimuth, H. C. and Fisher, R. S. (1958). Effect of pH and presence of other elements in solution on the absorption of boron. *J. invest. Derm.* **30**, 83–84.

Fricke, H. (1932). The theory of electrolytic polarization. *Phil. Mag.* **14**, 310–318.

Fry, P., Harkness, M. L. R., Harkness, R. D. and Nightingale, M. (1962). Mechanical properties of tissues of lathyritic animals. *J. Physiol.* **164**, 77–89.

Fujimori, B. (1955). Studies on the GSR using the current-and-potential method. *Jap. J. Physiol.* **5**, 394–405.

Gagge, A. P. (1937). A new physical variable associated with sensible and insensible perspiration. *Am. J. Physiol.* **120**, 277–287.

Gagge, A. P., Winslow, C.-E. A. and Herrington, L. P. (1938). Clothing and bodily reactions to temperature. *Am. J. Physiol.* **124**, 30–50.

Gasselt, H. R. M. and Vierhout, R. R. (1963). Registration of the insensible perspiration of small quantities of sweat. *Dermatologica* **127**, 255–259.

Gates, D. M. (1962). "Energy Exchange in the Biosphere." Harper and Ross, New York.

Gildemeister, M. (1928). Die Elektrizitätserzengung der Haut und der Drüsen. *In* Bethe, "Handbuch normalen pathologischen Physiologie" Bd VIII, Tl. 2, 766–777.

Gold, E. (1935). Effect of wind, temperature, humidity and sunshine on the loss of heat of a body at 98° F. *Q. Jl R. met. Soc.* **61**, 316–331.

Goldhamer, R. and Carson, S. (1963). Tracer procedure for the study of skin absorption. *J. Toilet Goods Ass.* **38**, 48–50.

Goldman, J., Hornby, P. and Long, C. (1964). Effect of the laser beam on the skin. *J. invest. Derm.* **42**, 231–234.

Goldman, L. and Cohen, C. (1963). Modification of the cellophane tape method for testing topical corticosteroids. *J. invest. Derm.* **41**, 101–102.

Goldman, L., Blaney, D. J., Kindel, D. J. and Franke, E. K. (1963). Effect of the laser beam on the skin. *J. invest. Derm.* **40**, 121–122.

Goldschmidt, S., McGlone, B. and Donal, J. S. (1934). Oxygen absorption through the skin. *Am. J. med. Sci.* **187**, 586–587.

Goldzieher, J. W. and Baker, R. E. (1960). The percutaneous absorption of estradiol 17β and progesterone. *J. invest. Derm.* **35**, 215–218.

Goldzieher, J. W., Roberts, J. S., Rawls, W. B. and Goldzieher, M. A. (1951). Chemical analysis of the intact skin by reflectance spectrophotometry. *Archs Derm. Syph.* **64**, 533–548.

Gougerot, L. (1947). Study of the impedance of skin to AC of low frequency during various dermatoses. *Annls Derm. Syph.* **7**, 101–111.

Gougerot, L. and Duvelleroy, M. (1960). Is the psychogalvanic reflex caused by rise of sweat in the ducts of the glands? *C. r. Séanc. Soc. Biol.* **154**, 2192.

Grant, R. T. (1935). Vascular reactions in the rabbit's ear. *Clin. Sci.* **2**, 1–26.

Gray, D. E. (1963). "American Institute of Physics Handbook", 2nd ed. Table 4g–12. McGraw-Hill, New York.

Griesemer, R. D. (1959). Protection against the transfer of matter through the skin. *In* "The Human Integument" (S. Rothman, ed.), pp. 25–46. American Association for the Advancement of Science Publication No. 54.

Grings, W. W. (1953). Methodological considerations underlying electrodermal measurement. *J. Psychol.* **35**, 271–282.

Grodstein, G. W. (1957). X-ray attenuation coefficients from 10 KeV to 100 MeV. U.S. natn. Bur. Stand. Circular 583.

Gross, J. (1950). A study of certain connective tissue constituents with the electron microscope. *Ann. N.Y. Acad. Sci.* **52**, 964–970.

Gross, J. and Schmitt, F. O. (1948). The structure of human skin collagen as studied with the electron microscope. *J. exp. Med.* **88**, 555–568.

Guibert, A. and Taylor, C. L. (1952). Radiation area of the human body. *J. appl. Physiol.* **5**, 24–37.

Hammel, H. T. (1955). Thermal properties of fur. *Am. J. Physiol.* **182**, 369–376.

Hammel, H. T. (1956). Infra-red emissivities of some Arctic fauna. *J. Mammal.* **37**, 375–378.

Hammel, H. T., Wyndham, C. H. and Hardy, J. D. (1958). Heat production and heat loss in the dog. *Am. J. Physiol.* **194**, 99–108.

Hancock, W., Whitehouse, A. G. R. and Haldane, J. S. (1929). Loss of water and salts through the skin. *Proc. R. Soc.* B, **105**, 43–59.

Hardy, J. D. (1949). Heat transfer. *In* "Physiology of Heat Regulation in the Science of Clothing" (L. H. Newburgh, ed.), p. 78. Saunders, Philadelphia.

Hardy, J. D. and Muschenheim, C. (1934). The emission, reflection and transmission of infra-red radiation by human skin. *J. clin. Invest.* **13**, 817–831.

Hardy, J. D. and Soderstrom, G. R. (1938). Heat loss and peripheral blood fiow. *J. Nutr.* **16**, 493–510.

Hardy, J. D., Hammel, H. T. and Murgatroyd, D. (1956). Spectral transmittance and reflectance of excised human skin. *J. appl. Physiol.* **9**, 257–264.

Harkness, M. L. R. and Harkness, R. D. (1959a). Effect of enzymes on mechanical properties of tissues. *Nature, Lond.* **183**, 1821–1822.

Harkness, M. L. R. and Harkness, R. D. (1959b). Changes in the physical properties of the uterine cervix of the rat during pregnancy. *J. Physiol.* **148**, 524-547.

Harkness, R. D. (1962). Biological functions of collagen. *Biol. Rev.* **36**, 399–463.

Harkness, R. D. (1964). Structure and metabolism of collagen. *In* "Progress in the Biological Sciences in Relation to Dermatology", 2nd ed. (A. Rook and R. H. Champion, eds.), pp. 3–24. Cambridge University Press, London.

Harkness, R. D. and Nightingale, M. (1962). Extensibility of the cervix uteri of the rat at different times of pregnancy. *J. Physiol.* **160**, 214–220.

Hart, J. S. (1956). Seasonal changes in insulation of fur. *Can. J. Zool.* **34**, 53–57.

Hart, J. S., Heroux, O., Cottle, W. H. and Mills, C. A. (1961). The influence of climate on metabolic and thermal responses of infant caribou. *Can. J. Zool.* **39**, 845–856.

Hartley, G. S. and Crank, J. (1949). Some fundamental definitions and concepts in diffusion. *Trans. Faraday Soc.* **45**, 801–818.

Harvey, R. A. (1954). Finger changes in monkeys following X-radiation, pp. 140–152; Effect of short wavelength radiations on human finger ridge detail, pp. 352–372. *In* "Biological Effects of External Radiation" (H. A. Blair, ed.). McGraw-Hill, New York.

Hatfield, H. S. (1950). A heat-flow meter. *J. Physiol.* **111**, 10–11P.

Hatfield, H. S. (1953). An apparatus for measuring the thermal conductivity of animal tissue. *J. Physiol.* **120**, 35–36P.

Hatfield, H. S. and Pugh, L. G. C. (1951). Thermal conductivity of human fat and muscle. *Nature, Lond.* **168**, 918–919.

Haurowitz, F. (1963). "The Chemistry and Function of Proteins," p. 140. Academic Press, New York.

Heerd, E. and Ohara, K. (1960). On the mechanism of water loss through human skin. *Pflüg. Arch. ges. Physiol.* **272**, 25.

Heerd, E. and Ohara, K. (1962). The relation of water loss through small skin areas in man to water vapour pressure, at normal skin temperature. *Pflüg. Arch. ges. Physiol.* **276**, 32–41.

Helde, M. and Seeberg, G. (1953). Cutaneous absorption studies using radio-phosphorus. *Acta derm.-vener.* **33**, 290–298.

Hendler, E., Crosbie, R. and Hardy, J. D. (1958). Measurement of heating of the skin during exposure to infra-red radiation. *J. appl. Physiol.* **12**, 177–185.

Henriques, F. C. and Moritz, A. R. (1947a). The conduction of heat to and through skin and the temperatures attained therein. *Am. J. Path.* **23**, 531–549.

Henriques, F. C. and Moritz, A. R. (1947b). The relative importance of time and surface temperature in the causation of cutaneous burns. *Am. J. Path.* **23**, 695–720.

Hensel, H. and Bender, F. (1956). Fortlanfende Bestimmung ger Hantdurchblutung am Menschen mit einem elektrischen Wärmeleitmesser. *Pflüg. Arch. ges. Physiol.* **263**, 603–614.

Hermann, F. and Prose, P. H. (1951). Studies on the quantity and replacement of ether-soluble substances on the human skin. *J. invest. Derm.* **16**, 217–230.

Hermann, F., Prose, P. H. and Sulzberger, M. B. (1952). The effect of sweat on the quantity of ether-soluble substances on the skin. *J. invest. Derm.* **21**, 397–417.

Herrington, L. P. (1940). The heat regulation of small laboratory animals at various environmental temperatures. *Am. J. Physiol.* **129**, 123–139.

Hertzmann, A. B. (1953). Some relations between skin temperature and blood flow. *Am. J. phys. Med.* **32**, 233–251.

Hertzmann, A. B. (1961). Effects of heat on the cutaneous blood flow. *Adv. Biol. Skin* **2**, 98–116.

Hertzmann, A. B. and Randall, W. C. (1948). Regional differences in the basal and maximal rates of blood flow in the skin. *J. appl. Physiol.* **1**, 234–241.

Higuchi, T. (1960). Physical chemical analysis of percutaneous absorption process from creams and ointments. *J. Soc. cosmet. Chem.* **11**, 85–96.

Higuchi, T. and Tillmann, W. J. (1961). Quantitative evaluation of the interaction of callus strips with some hydroxylic solvents. *J. invest. Derm.* **37**, 87–92.

Higuchi, T., Lueck, L. M., Wurster, D. E., Lemberger, A. P. and Busse, A. W. (1957). Investigation and development of protective ointments. *J. Am. pharm. Ass.* **46**, 694–701.

Hodge, H. C. and Sterner, J. H. (1943). The skin absorption of tricresyl phosphate. *J. Pharmac. exp. Ther.* **79**, 223–234.

Hodgman, C. D. (1963). "Handbook of Chemistry and Physics", 44th ed. Chemical Rubber Publishing Co., Cleveland, Ohio.

Holmes, A. W. (1961). A fatty acid-protein complex in human hair. *Nature, Lond.* **189**, 923.

Hongo, T. T. and Luck, C. P. (1953). The circulation in the tail of a monkey. *J. Physiol.* **122**, 570–581.

Horstmann, E. and Dabelow, A. (1957). "Handbuch der mikroskopischen Anatomie des Menchen: Haut und Sinnesorgane". Springer, Berlin.

Horstmann, E. and Knoop, A. (1958). Electron microscope studies of the epidermis. *Z. Zellforsch. mikrosk. Anat.* **47**, 348–362.

Howard-Flanders, P. (1958). Physical and chemical mechanisms in the injury of cells by ionising radiations. *Adv. biol. mec. Phys.* **6**, 553–603

Hulse, E. V. (1964). Biological effects of radiation on the skin—late effects. U.K. Atomic Energy Authority Report AHSB(RP)R39, pp. 21–27.

Hunter, R. and Williams, M. G. (1957). Studies of epidermal regeneration by means of a strip method. *J. invest. Derm.* **29**, 407–413.

Hurley, H. J. and Shelley, W. B. (1960). "The Human Apocrine Sweat Gland in Health and Disease." Thomas, Springfield.

Iampietro, P. F., Bass, D. E. and Buskirk, E. R. (1958). Heat exchanges of nude men in the cold. *J. appl. Physiol.* **12**, 351–356.

Ikeuchi, K. and Kuno, Y. (1927). On the regional differences of the perspiration on the surface of the body. *J. orient. Med.* **7**, 106–107.

Irving, L. (1956). Physiological insulation of swine as bare-skinned mammals. *J. appl. Physiol.* **9**, 414–420.

Irving, L. and Hart, J. S. (1957). The metabolism and insulation of seals as bare-skinned mammals in cold water. *Can. J. Zool.* **35**, 497–511.

Irving L. and Hart, J. S. (1959). The energetics of harbor seals in air and in water with special consideration of seasonal changes. *Can. J. Zool.* **37**, 447–457.

Irving, L. and Krog. J. (1954). Temperature of skin in the Arctic as a regulator of heat. *J. appl. Physiol.* **7**, 355–364.

Irving, L., Krog, J. and Monson, M. (1955). Metabolism of some Alaskan animals in winter and summer. *Physiol. Zöol.* **28**, 173–185.

Irving, L., Peyton, L. J. and Monson, M. (1956). Metabolism and insulation of swine as bare-skinned mammals. *J. appl. Physiol.* **9**, 421–426.

Irving, L., Schmidt-Nielsen, K. and Abrahamsen, N. S. B. (1957). The melting points of animal fats. *Physiol. Zöol.* **30**, 93–105.

Irving, L., Peyton, L. J., Bahn, C. H. and Peterson, R. S. (1962). Regulation of temperature in fur seals. *Physiol. Zöol.* **35**, 275–284.

Isherwood, P. A. (1963). A modified cell for the determination of water diffusion through skin. *J. invest. Derm.* **40**, 143–146.

Iunin, A. N. (1958). Speed and duration of sulphur penetration through animal skin. *Int. Abstr. med. Sci.* **14**, 2331.

Ive, H., Lloyd, J. and Magnus, I. A. (1965). Action spectra in idiopathic solar urticaria. *Br. J. Dermat.* **77**, 229–243.

Jacobson, W. (1953). Histological survey of normal connective tissue and its derivatives. *In* "Nature and Structure of Collagen" (J. T. Randall, ed.), pp. 6–13. Butterworth, London.

Jacquez, J. A. and Kuppenheim, H. F. (1954). Spectral reflectance of human skin in the region 235–1000 mμ. *J. appl. Physiol.* **7**, 523–528.

Jacquez, J. A. and Kuppenheim, H. F. (1955). Theory of the integrating sphere. *J. opt. Soc. Am.* **45**, 971–975.

Jacquez, J. A., Dimitroff, J. M. and Kuppenheim, H. F. (1955a). Spectral reflectance of the skin of rats and rabbits in the region 420–1000 mμ. *J. appl. Physiol.* **8**, 292–296.

Jacquez, J. A., Dimitroff, J. M. and Kuppenheim, H. F. (1955b). Spectral reflectance of human skin in the region 0·7–2·6 μ. *J. appl. Physiol.* **8**, 297–299.

Jacquez, J. A., Kuppenheim, H. F., Dimitroff, J. M., McKeehan, W. and Huss, J. (1955c). Spectral reflectance of human skin in the region 235–700 mμ. *J. appl. Physiol.* **8**, 212–214.

Jacquez, J. A., McKeehan, W., Huss, J., Dimitroff, J. M. and Kuppenheim, H. F. (1955d). Integrating sphere for the measurement of reflectance with the Beckman model DR recording spectrophotometer. *J. opt. Soc. Am.* **45**, 971–975.

Jarrett, A. (1958). The structure of collagen and elastic fibres in unprocessed skin. *Br. J. Derm.* **70**, 343.

Jelliffe, A. M. (1964). Biological effects of radiation on the skin—early effects. U.K. Atomic Energy Authority Report AHSB(RP)R39, pp. 10–21.

Johanssen, K. (1961). Temperature regulation in the armadillo. *Physiol. Zöol.* **34**, 126–144.

Jolly, H. W., Hailey, C. W. and Natick, J. (1961). pH Determination of the skin. *J. invest. Derm.* **36**, 305–308.

Jones, K. K., Spencer, M. C. and Sanchez, S. A. (1951). The estimation of rate of secretion of sebum in man. *J. invest. Derm.* **17**, 213–226.

Jores, A. (1930). Perspiratio insensibilis (1). *Z. exp. Med.* **71**, 170–185.

Jores, A. (1931). Perspiratio insensibilis (3). *Z. exp. Med.* **77**, 734–742.

Kahl, M. P. (1963). Thermoregulation in the wood stork with special reference to the role of the legs. *Physiol. Zöol.* **36**, 141–151.

Kaye, G. W. and Laby, T. H. (1958). "Tables of Physical and Chemical Constants", 12th ed. Longmans, Green, London.

Kayser, C. (1961). "Physiology of Natural Hibernation." Pergamon Press, London.

Kedem, O. and Katchalsky, A. (1961). A physical interpretation of the phenomenological coefficients of membrane permeability. *J. gen. Physiol.* **45**, 143–179.

Keller, P. (1931). Basal and tonic potentials across human skin. *Archs Derm. Syph.* **162**, 582–610.

Keller, R. (1958). Passage of bacteriophage particles through the intact skin of mice. *Science, N.Y.* **128**, 718–719.

Kerslake, D. McK., Brebner, D. F. and Waddell, J. D. (1956). The diffusion of water vapour through human skin. *J. Physiol.* **132**, 225–231.

Kibler, H. H. and Brody, S. (1952). Relative efficiency of surface evaporative, respiratory evaporative and non-evaporative cooling in relation to heat production in cattle, 0°–105° F. *Res. Bull. Mo. agric. Exp. Stn.* 497.

Kiistalla, V. and Mustakallio, K. K. (1964). *In-vivo* separation of epidermis by production of suction blisters. *Lancet* **1**, 1444–1445.

King, G. (1945). Permeability of keratin membranes to water vapour. *Trans. Faraday Soc.* **41**, 479–487.

Kirby-Smith, J. S., Blum, H. F. and Grady, H. G. (1942a). Penetration of ultra-violet radiation into skin as a factor in carcinogenesis. *J. natn. Cancer Inst.* **2**, 403–412.

Kirby-Smith, J. S., Blum, H. F. and Grady, H. G. (1942b). Quantitative induction of tumours in mice with ultra-violet radiation. *J. natn. Cancer Inst.* **2**, 259–268.

Kirk, E. (1948). Quantitative determination of the skin lipid secretion by middle-aged and old individuals. *J. Geront.* **3**, 251–266.

Kirk, E. and Kvorning, S. A. (1949). Quantitative measurements of the elastic properties of the skin and subcutaneous tissues in young and old individuals. *J. Geront.* **4**, 273–284.

Kirmiz, J. P. (1962). "Adaptation to Desert Environment." Butterworth, London.

Kjaersgaard, A. R. (1954). Perfusion of isolated dog skin, using the saphenous artery. *J. invest. Derm.* **22**, 135–141.

Kleiber, M. (1947). Body size and metabolic rate. *Physiol. Rev.* **27**, 511–541.

Kligman, A. M. (1963). The uses of sebum. *Br. J. Derm.* **75**, 307–319.

Klocke, R. A., Gurtner, G. H. and Farhi, L. E. (1963). Gas transfer across skin in man. *J. appl. Physiol.* **18**, 311–316.

Knapp, B. J. and Robinson, K. W. (1954). The role of water for heat dissipation by a Jersey cow and a Corriedale ewe. *Aust. J. agric. Res.* **5**, 568–577.

Kooynan, D. J. (1932). Lipids of the skin. *Archs Derm. Syph.* **25**, 444–450.

Kramer, H. and Little, V. (1953). The nature of reticulin. *In* "Nature and Structure of Collagen" (J. T. Randall, ed.), pp. 33–34. Butterworth, London.

Krause, R. A., Storz, H. and Voelkel, A. (1953). Direct current measurements of human skin. *Z. exp. Med.* **121**, 66–83.

Krogh, A. (1922). "The Anatomy and Physiology of Capillaries." Yale University Press, New Haven.

Kuno, Y. (1956). "Human Perspiration." Thomas, Springfield.

Kuppenheim, H. F. and Heer, R. R. (1952). Spectral reflectance of white and Negro skin between 440 and 1000 mμ. *J. appl. Physiol.* **4**, 800–806.

Kuppenheim, H. F., Dimitroff, J. M., Melotti, P. M., Graham, I. C. and Swanson, D. W. (1956). Spectral reflectance of the skin of Chester White pigs at 235–700 mμ and 0·707–2·6 μ. *J. appl. Physiol.* **9**, 75–78.

Ladell, W. S. S. (1945). Thermal sweating. *Br. med. Bull.* **3**, 175–178.

Laden, E. L., Gethner, P. and Erickson, J. O. (1957). Electron microscope study of keratohyalin in the formation of keratin. *J. invest. Derm.* **28**, 325–327.

Lagermalm, G. B., Philp, B. and Lindberg, J. (1951). Occurrence of thin membranes in the surface layers of human skin and in finger nails. *Nature, Lond.* **168**, 1080–1081.

Laurent, T., Ryan, M. and Pietruszkiewicz, A. (1960). Fractionation of hyaluronic acid. *Biochim. biophys. Acta* **42**, 476–485.

Lawler, J. C., Davis, M. J. and Griffith, E. C. (1960). The electrical impedance of the surface sheath of skin and deep tissues. *J. invest. Derm.* **34**, 301–308.

Lawson, A. W. (1964). Decontamination of the skin. U.K. Atomic Energy Authority Report, AHSB(RB)R39, 69–78.

Lentz, C. P. and Hart, J. S. (1960). The effect of wind and moisture on heat loss through the fur of the newborn caribou. *Can. J. Zool.* **38**, 679–688.

Lewis, T. and Zottermann, Y. (1927). The resistance of human skin to constant currents in relation to injury and vascular responses. *J. Physiol.* **62**, 280–288.

Linderstrom-Lang, K. and Duspiva, F. (1935). Keratin digestion in the larvae of the clothes moth. *Nature, Lond.* **135**, 1039–1040.

Lipkin, M. and Hardy, J. D. (1954). Measurement of some thermal properties of human tissue. *J. appl. Physiol.* **7**, 212–217.

Lizgunova, A. V. (1959). Penetration of micro-organisms through the skin of mice. *Bull. exp. Biol. Med. U.S.S.R.* **47**, 28.

Lloyd, D. P. C. (1960). Electrical impedance changes of the cat's foot pad in relation to sweat secretion and reabsorption. *J. gen. Physiol.* **43**, 713–722.

Lloyd, D. P. C. (1962). Secretion and reabsorption in eccrine sweat glands. *Adv. Biol. Skin* **3**, 127–151.

Lobitz, W. C. and Holyoke, J. B. (1954). The histochemical response of the human epidermis to controlled injury. *J. invest. Derm.* **22**, 189–198.

Loewenthal, L. J. A. and Pienaar, A. S. (1960). Elastosis and cutaneous irradiation injuries. *S. Afr. med. J.* **34**, 1076.

Loewi, G. (1961). The acid mucopolysaccharides of human skin. *Biochim. biophys. Acta* **52**, 435–440.

Loewi, G. and Meyer, K. (1958). The acid mucopolysaccharides of embryonic skin. *Biochim. biophys. Acta* **27**, 453–456.

Lorincz, A. L. (1960). Physiological and pathological changes in skin from sunburn and suntan. *J. Am. med. Ass.* **173**, 1227–1231.

Lotmar, R. (1958). Über die Anwedung der Isotopenmethode in der Balneologie. *Dt. med. Wschr.* **83**, 218–221.

Lovatt-Evans, C. (1945). "Principles of Human Physiology", p. 769. Churchill, London.

Love, L. H. (1949). Heat loss and blood flow of the feet under hot and cold conditions. *J. appl. Physiol.* **1**, 20–34.

Loveday, D. E. (1961). An *in vitro* method for studying percutaneous absorption. *J. Soc. cosmet. Chem.* **12**, 224–239.

Lucas, N. S. (1930). The permeability of human epidermis to ultra-violet radiation. *Biochem. J.* **25**, 57–70.

Luck, C. P. and Wright, P. G. (1959). The skin secretion of the hippopotamus (T). *J. Physiol.* **148**, 22P.

Lundgren, H. P. and Ward, W. H. (1963). The keratins. *In* "Ultrastructure of Protein Fibres" (R. Borysko, ed.), pp. 39–122. Academic Press, New York.

McDowell, R. E., Lee, D. M. K. and Fohrman, M. H. (1954). The measurement of water evaporation from limited areas of a normal body surface. *J. Anim. Sci.* **13**, 405–416.

MacFarlane, W. V., Morris, R. J. and Howard, B. (1956). Water economy of tropical merino sheep. *Nature, Lond,* **178**, 304–305.

Mackee, G. M., Sulzberger, M. B., Hermann, F. and Baer, R. B. L. (1945). Histologic studies on percutaneous penetration. *J. invest. Derm.* **6**, 43–61.

Mackenna, R. M. B., Wheatley, V. R. and Wormall, A. (1950). The composition of the surface skin fat from the human forearm. *J. invest. Derm.* **15**, 33–47.

McKenzie, A. W. and Stoughton, R. B. (1962). Methods for comparing percutaneous absorption of steroids. *Archs Derm.* **85**, 608–610.

McLean, D. and Hale, C. W. (1941). Studies on diffusing factors. *Biochem. J.* **35**, 159–183.

McLean, J. A. (1963). Measurement of cutaneous moisture vaporization from cattle by ventilated capsules. *J. Physiol.* **167**, 417–426.

Magnus, I. A. (1964). Studies with a monochromator in the common idiopathic photodermatoses. *Br. J. Derm.* **76**, 245–264.

Magnus, I. A. and Porter, A. D. (1959). A case of urticaria solaris studied with a monochromator. *Br. J. Derm.* **71**, 51–60.

Mali, J. W. H. (1955). The transport of water through the human epidermis. *J. invest. Derm.* **27**, 451–469.

Mali, J. W. H., van Kooten, W. J. and van Neer, F. C. J. (1963). Some aspects of the behaviour of chromium compounds in the skin. *J. invest. Derm.* **41**, 111–122.

Malkinson, F. D. (1958). Studies on the percutaneous absorption of C-14 labelled steriods by use of the gas flow cell. *J. invest. Derm.* **31**, 19–26.

Malkinson, F. D. (1960). Percutaneous absorption of adrenal steroids. *J. Soc. cosmet. Chem.* **11**, 146–159.

Malkinson, F. D. and Rothman, S. (1962). Percutaneous absorption. *In* "Handbuch der Haut" (E. Jadassohn, ed.), Vol. 1, pp. 90–156. Springer, Berlin.

Martin, C. J. (1930). Thermal adjustment of man and animals to external conditions. *Lancet* **1**, 673–678.

Marzulli, F. N. (1962). Barriers to skin penetration. *J. invest. Derm.* **37**, 387–393.

Marzulli, F. N. and Callahan, J. F. (1957). The capacity of certain common laboratory animals to sweat. *J. Am. vet. Med. Ass.* **131**, 80–81.

Marzulli, F. N. and Tregear, R. T. (1961). Identification of a barrier layer in skin. *J. Physiol.* **157**, 52–53P.

Matoltsy, A. G. (1958). The chemistry of keratinization. *In* "The Biology of Hair Growth" (W. Montagna and R. A. Ellis, eds.), pp. 135–170. Academic Press, New York.

Matoltsy, A. G., Matoltsy, M. and Schragger, A. (1962). Observations on the regenerating skin barrier. *J. invest. Derm.* **38**, 251–253.

Maurice, D. M. and Mishima, S. (1961). The effect of normal evaporation on the eye. *Expl. Eye Res.* **1**, 46–52.

Mercer, E. H. (1962). "Keratin and Keratinization." Pergamon Press, Oxford.

Meyer, F. and Kerk, L. (1959). A comparative study of the permeability of skin to aliphatic media. *Rauryn-Schmiedebergs Arch. exp. Path. Pharmak.* **235**, 267–278.

Meyer, K. and Chaffee, E. (1941). Mucopolysaccharides of skin. *J. biol. Chem.* **138**, 491.

Mitchell, J. S. (1938). The origin of the erythema curve and the pharmacological action of ultraviolet radiation. *Proc. R. Soc.,* B, **126**, 241–246.

Mole, R. H. (1948). Relative humidity of skin. *J. Physiol.* **107**, 399–411.

Molnar, G. W. and Rosenbaum, J. C. (1963). Surface temperature measurement with thermocouples. *In* "Temperature: its Measurement and Control in Science and Industry" (J. D. Hardy, ed.), vol. 3, pp. 3–13. Reinhold, New York.

Monash, S. (1957). Location of the superficial barrier to skin penetration. *J. invest. Derm.* **29**, 367–376.

Monash, S. and Blank, H. (1958). Location and reformation of the epithelial barrier to water vapour. *Archs Derm.* **78**, 710–714.

Montagna, W. (1962). "The Structure and Function of Skin." Academic Press, New York.

Montagna, W. (1963). Comparative aspects of sebaceous glands. *Adv. Biol. Skin* **4**, 32–45.

Montagna, W., Ellis, R. A. and Silver, A. F. (1962). Eccrine sweat glands and eccrine sweating. *Adv. Biol. Skin* **3**.

Montagu, J. D. (1958). The psychogalvanic reflex: comparison of AC skin resistance and skin potential changes. *J. neurol. neurosurg. Psychiat.* **21**, 119–128.

Morton, J. H., Kingsley, H. D. and Pearse, H. E. (1952). Studies on threshold flash burns. *Surg. Gynec. Obstet.* **94**, 317–322.

Moss, K. N. (1923). Some effects of high air temperatures and muscular exertion upon colliers. *Proc. R. Soc.* B, **95**, 181–200.

Mount, L. E. (1959). The metabolic rate of the newborn pig in relation to environmental temperature and to age. *J. Physiol.* **147**, 333–345.

Mount, L. E. (1962). Evaporative heat loss in the newborn pig. *J. Physiol.* **164**, 274–281.

Mount, L. E. (1965). The young pig and its physical environment. *In* "Energy Metabolism" (K. L. Blaxter, ed.), pp. 379–385. Academic Press, London.

Muir, H. (1964). Mucopolysaccharides in the dermis. *In* "Progress in the Biological Sciences in Relation to Dermatology" (A. Rook and R. H. Champion, eds.), pp. 25–36. Cambridge University Press, London.

Namba, T. and Hiraki, K. (1958). PAM therapy for alkyl phosphate poisoning. *J. Am. med. Ass.* **166**, 1834–1839.

Naylor, P. F. D. (1959). The polarographic measurement of oxygen tension. *J. Physiol.* **145**, 3P.

Negherbon, W. O. (1959). "Handbook of Toxicology." Vol 3. Insecticides. Wright Air Development Center Report, pp. 55–56.

Neumann, R. E. and Logan, M. A. (1950). The determination of collagen and elastin in tissues. *J. biol. Chem.* **186**, 549–556.

Newbery, G. R. (1964). Measurement and assessment of skin doses from skin contamination. U.K. Atomic Energy Authority Rep. AHSB(RP)R39, pp. 44–53.

Nicolaides, N. (1961). Chromatographic analysis of the waxes of human scalp skin surface fat. *J. invest. Derm.* **37**, 507–511.

Nicolaides, N. and Wells, G. C. (1957). On the biosynthesis of the free fatty acids in human skin surface fat. *J. invest. Derm.* **29**, 429–432.

Norgaard, O. (1957). Investigations with radioactive nickel, cobalt and chromium. *Acta derm.-vener.* **37**, 440–445.

Odland, G. F. (1958). The fine structure of the inter-relationship of cells in the human epidermis. *J. biophys. biochem. Cytol.* **4**, 529–538.

Odland, G. F. (1960). A submicroscopic granular component in human epidermis. *J. invest. Derm.* **34,** 11–15.

Ogston, A. G. and Stanier, J. E. (1953). The physiological function of hyaluronic acid in synovial fluid. *J. Physiol.* **119,** 244–252.

Onken, H. D. and Moyer, C. A. (1963). The water barrier in human epidermis. *Archs Derm.* **87,** 584–590.

Oppel, T. W. and Hardy, J. D. (1937). A comparison of the sensation produced by infra-red and visible radiation. *J. clin. Invest.* **16,** 517–524.

Pappenheimer, J. R. (1953). Passage of molecules through blood vessel walls. *Physiol. Rev.* **33,** 387–423.

Partington, M. W. (1954). The vascular response of the skin to ultraviolet light. *Clin. Sci.* **13,** 425–439.

Pasquill, F. (1949). Eddy diffusion of water vapour and heat near the ground. *Proc. R. Soc.* A, **198,** 116–140.

Passow, H. (1964). Passive ion permeability. Abstracts of the International Biophysical Congress, Paris.

Pathak, M. A. (1962). Mechanism of psoralen photosensitization and *in vivo* biological action spectrum of 8-methoxypsoralen. *J. invest. Derm.* **37,** 397–407.

Pauly, H. (1962). Electrical proporties of the cytoplasmic membrane and the cytoplasm of bacteria and protoplasts. *Bio-Medical Electronics* **9,** 93–95.

Pearce, R. H. and Watson, E. M. (1949). The mucopolysaccharides of human skin. *Can. J. Res.* **27E,** 43.

Pearse, A. G. E. (1960). "Histochemistry, Theoretical and Applied", p. 228. Churchill, London.

Pearson, A. R. and Gair, C. J. D. (1931). Penetration of radiation into animal tissues. *Br. J. phys. Med.* **6,** 27–30.

Pearson, R. W. and Spargo, B. (1962). Electron microscope studies of dermo-epidermal separation in human skin. *J. invest. Derm.* **36,** 213–224.

Pennes, H. H. (1949). Analysis of tissue and arterial blood temperatures in the resting human forearm. *J. appl. Physiol.* **1,** 93–122.

Petit, E. (1932). Measurement of ultraviolet solar radiation. *Astrophys. J.* **75,** 185–221.

Petrun, N. M. (1961). Percutaneous respiration in children of various ages. *Sechenov Physiol. J.* **47,** 1025–1027. (Trans.)

Pinkus, H. (1952). Biometric data on regeneration of the human epidermis after stripping. *J. invest. Derm.* **19,** 431–446.

Pinkus, H. (1954). The biology of epidermal cells. *In* "Physiology and Biochemistry of the Skin" (S. Rothman, ed.), pp. 554–600. Chicago University Press.

Pinson, E. A. (1942). Evaporation from human skin with sweat glands inactivated. *Am. J. Physiol.* **187,** 492–503.

Plutchik, R. and Hirsch, H. R. (1963). Skin impedance and phase angle as a function of frequency and current. *Science, N.Y.* **141,** 926–928.

Polyakova, T. I. (1962). A study of the cornification of the cutaneous epithelium of the lizard. *Dokl. Akad. Nauk.* **142,** 122. (Trans.)

Ponder, E. (1961). Thermal conductivity of blood and of various tissues. *J. gen. Physiol.* **45,** 545–551.

Pratt, A. W. (1962). Heat transfer in porous materials. *Research* **15,** 214–223.

Prouty, L. R. (1949). Heat loss and heat production of cats at different environmental temperatures. *Fedn Proc. Fedn Am. Socs exp. Biol.* **8**, 128–129.

Pryor, M. (1952). Rheology of muscle. *In* "Deformation and Flow in Biological Systems" (A. Frey-Wyssling, ed.), pp. 157–193. North Holland, Publishing Co., Amsterdam.

Ramanathan, N., Sikorski, J. and Woods, H. J. (1955). The surface structure of wool fibres. *Proc. int. Wool Textile Res. Cong.* Vol. F, pp. 63–91. Commonwealth Scientific and Industrial Research Organization, Melbourne.

Reader, S. R. (1952). The effective thermal conductivity of normal and rheumatic tissues in response to cooling. *Clin. Sci.* **11**, 1–12.

Rein, H. (1924). Electro-endosmosis in excised human skin. *Z. Biol.* **81**, 125–140.

Rein, H. (1926). Current flow and electromotive force across human skin. *Z. Biol.* **85**, 195–247.

Richardson, H. B. (1926). The effect of the absence of sweat glands on the elimination of water from the skin and lung. *J. biol. Chem.* **67**, 397–411.

Richter, C. P. (1946). Instructions for using the cutaneous resistance recorder on peripheral nerve injuries, sympathectomies and paravertebral blocks. *J. Neurosurg.* **3**, 181–191.

Richter, C. P. and Whelan, F. (1943). Sweat gland responses to sympathetic stimulation studied by the galvanic skin reflex method. *J. Neurophysiol.* **6**, 191–194.

Richter, C. P., Woodruff, B. G. and Eaton, B. C. (1943). Hand and foot patterns of low electrical skin resistance. *J. Neurophysiol.* **6**, 417–424.

Riek, R. F. and Lee, D. H. K. (1948). Reactions to hot atmospheres of Jersey cows in milk. *J. Dairy Res.* **15**, 219–226.

Riemerschmid, G. and Elder, J. S. (1945). Absorptivity for solar radiation of different coloured hairy coats of cattle. *Onderstepoort J. vet. Sci.* **20**, 223–234.

Roberts, J. K. and Miller, A. R. (1951). "Heat and Thermodynamics." Blackie, London.

Robinson, S. and Gerking, S. D. (1947). Thermal balance of men working in extreme heat. *Am. J. Physiol.* **149**, 476–488.

Robinson, S. and Robinson, A. H. (1954). Chemical composition of sweat. *Physiol. Rev.* **34**, 202–220.

Roeder, F. (1934). Die Messung der Wärmeleitzahl der menschlichen Haut und ihre Veränderlichkeit. *Z. Biol.* **95**, 164–168.

Rogers, G. E. and Filshie, B. K. (1963). Some aspects of the ultrastructure of α-keratin, bacterial flagella and feather keratin. *In* "Ultrastructure of Protein Fibers" (R. Borasky, ed.), pp. 123–138. Academic Press, New York.

Rollhauser, H. (1950). The tensile strength of human skin. *Gegenbauers morph. Jb.* **90**, 249–261.

Ropes, M. W., Robertson, W. V. B., Rossmeisl, E., Peabody, R. B. and Bauer, W. (1947). Synovial fluid mucin. *Acta med. scand.* **196**, 700.

Rosendal, T. (1943). Studies on the conducting properties of the human skin to direct current. *Acta physiol. scand.* **5**, 130–151.

Rosendal, T. (1944). Further studies on the conducting properties of human skin to DC and AC. *Acta physiol. scand.* **8**, 183–202.

Rosendal, T. (1945). Concluding studies on the conducting properties of human skin to AC. *Acta physiol. scand.* **9**, 39–49.

Rothman, S. (1954). "Physiology and Biochemistry of the Skin." Chicago University Press.

Rottier, P. B. and van der Leun, J. C. (1960). Hyperaemia of the deeper cutaneous vessels after irradiation of human skin with large doses of visible and ultraviolet light. *Br. J. Derm.* **72**, 591-606.

Rubin, S. H. (1960). Percutaneous absorption of vitamins. *J. Soc. cosmet. Chem.* **11**, 160–169.

Rudall, K. M. and Durward, A. (1958). The vascularity and patterns of growth of hair follicles. *In* "The Biology of Hair Growth" (W. Montagna and R. A. Ellis, eds.), pp. 189–218. Academic Press, New York.

Rutenfranz, J. and Wenzel, H. G. (1958). Quantitative relationship between water output, alternating current resistance and capacity of the skin during work and at different room temperatures. *Int. Z. Physiol.* **17**, 155–176.

Ryder, M. L. (1955). The blood supply to the wool follicle. *Proc. Int. Wool Textile Res. Conf.* Vol. F, 63–91. Commonwealth Scientific and Industrial Research Organization, Melbourne.

Ryder, M. L. (1964). Moulting and hair replacement. *In* "Progress in the Biological Sciences in Relation to Dermatology", 2nd ed. (A. Rook and R. H. Champion, eds.), pp. 325–336. Cambridge University Press, Cambridge.

Schade, H. (1912). Die Elastizitatsfunktion des Bindegewebes und die initiale Messung ihrer Storungen. *Z. exp. Path. Ther.* **11**, 369–399.

Scheuplein, R. J. (1964). A survey of some fundamental aspects of the absorption and reflection of light by tissue. *J. Soc. cosmet. Chem.* **15**, 111–122.

Schirren, C. G. (1955). pH Values on the skin surface. *J. invest. Derm.* **24**, 485–487.

Schmidt-Nielsen, K. (1946). Melting-points of human fats as related to their location in the body. *Acta physiol. scand.* **12**, 123–129.

Schmidt-Nielsen, K. (1954). Heat regulations in small and large desert mammals. *In* "Biology of Deserts", pp. 182–187. Institute of Biology, London.

Schmidt-Nielsen, K., Schmidt-Nielsen, B., Jarnum, S. A. and Houpt, T. R. (1957). Body temperature of the camel and its water economy. *Am. J. Physiol.* **188**, 103–117.

Schmitt, F. O., Hall, C. E. and Jakus, M. A. (1942). Electron microscopic investigations of the structure of collagen. *J. cell. comp. Physiol.* **20**, 11–33.

Schmitt, F. O., Gross, J. and Highberger, J. H. (1955). States of aggregation of collagen. *Symp. Soc. exp. Biol.* **9**, 148.

Scholander, P. F. (1955). Climatic adaptation in homoeotherms. *Evolution* **9**, 15–26.

Scholander, P. F. and Krog, J. (1957). Countercurrent heat exchange and vascular bundles in sloths. *J. appl. Physiol.* **10**, 405–411.

Scholander, P. F. and Schevill, W. E. (1955). Countercurrent vascular heat exchange in the fins of whales. *J. appl. Physiol.* **8**, 279–282.

Scholander, P. R., Walters, V., Hock, R. and Irving, L. (1950a). Body insulation of some tropical and Arctic mammals and birds. *Biol. Bull. mar. biol. Lab., Woods Hole* **99**, 225–236.

Scholander, P. R., Walters, V., Hock, R., Irving, L. and Johnson, F. (1950b). Heat regulation in some Arctic and tropical mammals and birds. *Biol. Bull. mar. biol. lab., Woods Hole* **99**, 237–258.

Scholander, P. R., Walters, V., Hock, R. and Irving, L. (1950c). Adaptation of Arctic and tropical mammals and birds in relation to body temperature and insulation. *Biol. Bull. mar. biol. Lab., Woods Hole* **99**, 259–271.

Scholander, P. F., Hammel, H. T., Hart, J. S., LeMessurier, D. H. and Steen, J. (1958a). Cold adaptation in Australian aborigines. *J. appl. Physiol.* **13**, 211–218.

Scholander, P. F., Hammel, H. T., Anderssen, K. L. and Loyning, Y. (1958b). Metabolic acclimation in man. *J. appl. Physiol.* **12**, 1–8.

Schwan, H. P. (1963). Determination of biological impedances. "Physical Techniques in Biological Research" (W. L. Nastuk, ed.), Vol. 6, pp. 323–408. Academic Press, New York.

Scott, A. and Kalz, F. (1956). The penetration and distribution of hydrocortisone in human skin after its application. *J. invest. Derm.* **26**, 149–158.

Selby, C. C. (1957). Electron microscopy of human epidermis. *J. invest. Derm.* **29**, 131–149.

Shelley, W. B. (1954). The effect of poral closure on the secretory function of the eccrine sweat gland. *J. invest. Derm.* **22**, 267–271.

Shelley, W. B. and Melton, F. M. (1949). Factors accelerating the penetration of histamine through normal intact skin. *J. invest. Derm.* **13**, 61–71.

Side, H. J. A. and Rudall, K. M. (1964). Rates of hair growth. *In* "Progress in the Biological Sciences in Relation to Dermatology", 2nd ed. (A. Rook and R. H. Champion, eds.), pp. 337–354. Cambridge University Press, London.

Siple, P. A. and Passel, C. F. (1945). Dry atmospheric cooling in subfreezing temperatures. *Proc. Am. Phil. Soc.* **89**, 177–199.

Smith, J. G., Davidson, E. A. and Clark, R. D. (1962). Hexosamine content of keratinous structures. *Fedn. Proc. Fedn. Am. Socs. exp. Biol.* **21**, 172.

Smith, Q. T. (1964). Body weight, cutaneous collagen and hexosamine of cortisone-treated female rats of various ages. *J. invest. Derm.* **42**, 353–358.

Snyder, F. H. (1960). Systemic toxicological reactions resulting from percutaneous absorption. *J. Soc. cosmet. Chem.* **11**, 117–126.

Soffen, G. A. and Blum, H. F. (1961). Quantitative measurements of changes in mouse skin following a single dose of ultraviolet light. *J. cell. comp. Physiol.* **58**, 81–110.

Speakman, J. B. (1955). The chemistry of keratinous structures. *Symp. Soc. exp. Biol.* **2**, 169–182.

Spier, H. W. and Pascher, G. (1956). On the analytical and functional physiology of the skin surface. *Hautarzt* **7**, 55–60.

Spiers, F. W. (1946). Effective atomic number and energy absorption in tissues. *Br. J. Radiol.* **19**, 52–63.

Stahl, W. H., McQue, B., Mandels, G. R. and Siu, G. H. (1950). Studies on the microbiological degradation of wool. *Text. Res. J.* **20**, 570–579.

Staverman, A. J. (1954). The physics of the phenomenon of permeability. *Acta physiol. pharmac. néerl.* **3**, 522–535.

Steigleder, G. K. and Raab, W. P. (1962). Skin protection provided by ointments. *J. invest. Derm.* **38**, 129–131.

Stevanovic, D. V. (1960). Sun screening substances. *Br. J. Derm.* **72**, 271–278.

Stewart, R. E., Pickett, E. E. and Brody, S. (1951). Effect of increasing temperature from 65°–95° F on the reflection of visible radiation from the hair of Brown Swiss and Brahman cows. *Res. Bull. Mo. Agric. Exp. Stn* 484.

Stoughton, R. B. and Cronin, E. (1962). Regional variation and the effect of hydration and epidermal stripping on percutaneous absorption. *Br. J. Derm.* **74**, 265–272.

Stoughton, R. B. and Cronin, E. (1963). Nicotinic acid and ethyl nicotinate in excised human skin. *Archs Derm.* **87**, 445–449.

Stoughton, R. B. and Fritsch, W. C. (1963). The effect of temperature and humidity on the penetration of acetylsalicylic acid in excised human skin. *J. invest. Derm.* **41**, 307–312.

Stoughton, R. B., Clendenning, W. E. and Kruse, D. (1960). Percutaneous absorption of nicotinic acid and its derivatives. *J. invest. Derm.* **35**, 337–342.

Strauss, J. S. and Pochi, P. E. (1961). The quantitative gravimetric determination of sebum production. *J. invest. Derm.* **36**, 293–298.

Strauss, J., Kligman, A. M. and Greenberg, S. (1954). Influence of anoxia on the depilation of mouse hair with X-rays. *J. invest. Derm.* **22**, 129–134.

Stüpel, H. and Szakall, A. (1957). "Die Wirkung von Waschmitteln auf die Haut." Huthig, Heidelberg.

Stuttgen, A. and Betzler, H. (1956). On the penetration of electrolytes (calcium, sulphate and phosphate) into mouse skin. *Arch. klin. exp. Derm.* **203**, 472.

Suchi, T. (1955). Experiments on electrical resistance of the human epidermis. *Jap. J. Physiol.* **5**, 75–80.

Swanbeck, G. (1959). Macromolecular organization of epidermal keratin. *Acta derm.-vener.* **39**, Suppl. 43.

Szabo, G. (1962). The number of eccrine sweat glands in human skin. *Adv. Biol. Skin.* **3**, 1–5.

Szakall, A. (1955). Die H-ionenkonzentration bestimmenden Wirkstoffe in der Epidermis. *Arch. klin. exp. Derm.* **201**, 331–360.

Takagi, K. and Nakayama, T. (1958). Two components involved in the galvanic skin response. *Jap. J. Physiol.* **8**, 21–30.

Takagi, K. and Nakayama, T. (1959). Peripheral effector mechanism of galvanic skin reflex. *Jap. J. Physiol.* **9**, 1–7.

Takagi, S. and Tagawa, M. (1956). A note on the shape and size of the human eccrine sweat pore. *Jap. J. Physiol.* **6**, 47–49.

Takenaka, T. (1963). Effect of temperature and metabolic inhibitors on the active sodium transport in frog skin. *Jap. J. Physiol.* **13**, 208.

Taneja, G. C. (1959). Cutaneous evaporative loss measured from limited areas and its relationship with skin, rectal and air temperatures. *J. agric. Sci.* **52**, 62–65.

Tas, J. and Feige, Y. (1958). Penetration of radio-iodide through human skin. *J. invest. Derm.* **30**, 193–197.

Taylor, D. M. (1961). A new instrument for measuring the galvanic skin response. D.S.I.R. Res. Note RN 3952.

Taylor, E. A. (1961). Oil adsorption: a method for determining the affinity of skin to adsorb oil from aqueous dispersion. *J. invest. Derm.* **37**, 69–72.

Teorell, T. (1964). Unstable phenomena in membranes. Abstracts of the International Biophysics Congress, Paris.

Thomas, P. E. and Korr, I. M. (1957). Relationship between sweat gland activity and electrical resistance of the skin. *J. appl. Physiol.* **10**, 505–510.

Thompson, N. (1962). Eccrine sweat glands in human skin grafts. *Adv. Biol. Skin* **3**, 76–96.

Thomson, M. L. (1955). Relative efficiency of pigment and horny layer thickness in protecting the skin of Europeans and Africans against solar ultraviolet radiation. *J. Physiol.* **127**, 236–246.

Towler, G. S. (1954). The use of barrier creams for hand protection against radioactive contamination. *Chemy Ind.*, 387.

Tregear, R. T. (1960). Epidermis as a thick membrane. *J. Physiol.* **153**, 54–55P.

Tregear, R. T. (1961). Relative penetrability of hair follicles and epidermis. *J. Physiol.* **156**, 303–313.

Tregear, R. T. (1962). The structures which limit the penetrability of skin. *J. Soc. cosmet. Chem.* **13**, 145–151.

Tregear, R. T. (1964a). Skin permeability and radioactive contamination. U.K. Atomic Energy Auth. Res. Rep. AHSB(RP) R39, 79–85.

Tregear, R. T. (1964b). The permeability of skin to molecules of widely differing properties. *In* "Progress in Biological Science in Relation to Dermatology" (A. J. Rook, ed.), Vol. 2. Cambridge University Press, London.

Tregear, R. T. (1965a). Hair density, wind speed and heat loss. *J. appl. Physiol.* **20**, 796–801.

Tregear, R. T. (1965b). The interpretation of skin impedance measurements. *Nature, Lond.* **205**, 600–601.

Tregear, R. T. (1966a). The permeability of mammalian skin to ions. *J. invest. Derm.* **46**, 16–23.

Tregear, R. T. (1966b). The permeability of skin to albumin, dextrans and polyvinyl pyrrolodone. *J. invest. Derm.* **46**, 24–27.

Tregear, R. T. and Dirnhuber, P. (1962). The mass of keratin removed from the stratum corneum by stripping with adhesive tape. *J. invest. Derm.* **38**, 375–381.

Tregear, R. T. and Dirnhuber, P. (1965). Viscous flow in compressed human and rat skin. *J. invest. Derm.* **45**, 119–125.

Treherne, J. E. (1956). Permeability of skin to some non-electrolytes. *J. Physiol.* **133**, 171–180.

Tui, C., Kuo, N. H. and Simuangco, S. (1949). Studies on scleroderma. *J. invest. Derm.* **15**, 117–118.

Tunbridge, R. E., Tattersall, R. N., Hall, D. A., Astbury, W. T. and Read, R. (1952). The fibrous structure of normal and abnormal human skin. *Clin. Sci.* **11**, 315–323.

Tunbridge, R. E. (1964). The ageing of connective tissue. *In* "Progress in the Biological Sciences in Relation to Dermatology", 2nd ed. (A. J. Rook and R. H. Champion, eds.), pp. 67–76. Cambridge University Press, London.

Tuwiner, S. B. (1962). "Diffusion and Membrane Technology." Reinhold, New York.

Valette, G., Cavier, R. and Savel, J. (1954). Percutaneous absorption and chemical constitution: hydrocarbons, alcohols and esters. *Archs int. Pharmacodyn. Thér.* **97**, 232–240.

Vandekar, M., Komanov, I. and Kobrehel, D. (1963). Study of the dermal toxicity of organophosphorus compounds. *Arh. Hig. Rada* **14**, 7–18.

Vennart, J. (1954). Some physical measurements in the Grenz ray region. *Br. J. Radiol.* **27**, 524–531.

Vickers, C. (1964). The role of the epidermis as a reservoir for topically applied agents. *In* "Progress in the Biological Sciences in Relation to Dermatology" (A. J. Rook, ed.), Vol. 2. Cambridge University Press, London.

Vinson, L. J. and Choman, B. R. (1960). Percutaneous absorption and surface-active agents. *J. Soc. cosmet. Chem.* **11**, 127–137.

Volkmann, R. (1950). Versuche zur Feststellung der Erneurungsdauer geschichteter Plattenepithelien. *Anat. Nachr.* **1**, 86–88.

Wahlberg, J. E. and Skog, E. (1962). Percutaneous absorption of mercuric chloride in guinea pigs. *Acta derm.-vener.* **42**, 418–425.

Wahlberg, J. E. and Skog, E. (1963). The percutaneous absorption of sodium chromate in the guinea pig. *Acta derm.-vener.* **43**, 102–108.

Wahlberg, J. E., Skog, E. and Friberg, L. (1961). Absorption of mercuric chloride and methyl mercury dicyandiamide in guinea-pigs through normal and pre-treated skin. *Acta derm.-vener.* **41**, 40–52.

Ward, J. S., Bredell, G. A. C. and Wenzel, H. G. (1960). Responses of Bushmen and Europeans to winter night temperatures in the Kalahari. *J. appl. Physiol.* **15**, 667–670.

Washburn, E. W. (1929). "International Critical Tables." McGraw-Hill, New York.

Weinstein, G. D. and Boucek, R. J. (1960). Collagen and elastin of human dermis. *J. invest. Derm.* **35**, 227–230.

Welbourn, E. (1964). The arteriovenous anastamoses of the skin. *In* "Progress in the Biological Sciences in Relation to Dermatology", 2nd ed. (A. Rook and R. H. Champion, eds.), pp. 391–402. Cambridge University Press, London.

Wells, A. C. (1957). The cellophane tape method. *Br. J. Derm.* **69**, 11–18.

Wells, F. V. and Lubowe, I. I. (1964). "Cosmetics and the Skin", pp. 262–273. Reinhold, New York.

Wenzel, H. G. (1948). Study of the tearing and stretching of skin. *Zentbl. allg. Path. path. Anat.* **85**, 117–118.

Wepierre, J. (1963). Etude quantitative de la pénétration percutanée chez la souris d'un solvant lipophile, le p-cymène. *C. r. hebd. Séanc. Acad. Sci., Paris* **256**, 1628–1630.

Wepierre, J. and Valette, G. (1962). La traversée de la barrière lipidique cutanée chez le chien par un solvant lipophile, le p-cymène. *C. r. hebd. Séanc. Acad. Sci., Paris* **254**, 2092–2094.

Wheatley, V. R. and Reinartson, R. P. (1959). Studies on the chemical composition of human epidermal lipids. *J. invest. Derm.* **32**, 49–60.

Wheatley, V. R., Coon, W. M., Herrmann, F. and Mandol, L. (1963). Free fatty acids of the skin surface in normal and abnormal keratinisation. *J. invest. Derm.* **41**, 259–264.

Whittow, G. C. (1962). The significance of the extremities of the ox in thermoregula-tion. *J. agric. Sci.* **58**, 109–120.

Wilcott, R. C. (1962). Effects of partial puncture of the epidermis on skin resistance and skin potential. *Psychol. Rep.* **10**, 27–32.

Wildman, A. B. (1954). "The Microscopy of Animal Textile Fibres." Wool Industry Research Association, Leeds.

Wislocki, G. B. (1928). Gross and microscopic anatomy of sloths. *J. Morph.* **46**, 317–377.

Wislocki, G. B. and Enders, R. K. (1935). Body temperature of sloths, anteaters and armadillos. *J. Mammal.* **16**, 328–329.

Wislocki, G. B. and Straus, W. L. (1932). On the blood vascular bundles in the limbs of certain edentates and lemurs. *Bull. Mus. comp. Zool. Harv.* **74**, 1–15.

Wolf, J. (1937). The contours of the human skin surface. *Bull. int. Acad. Sci. Boheme* 1937, 1–12.

Wolf, J. (1954). Das relief des geschichten Plattenepithel. *Ceskoslov. Morf.* **2**, 49–61.

Wurster, D. E. and Kramer, S. F. (1961). Investigation of some factors influencing percutaneous absorption. *J. Pharm. Sci.* **50**, 288–293.

Yokota, T. and Fujimori, B. (1962). Impedance change of the skin during the galvanic skin reflex. *Jap. J. Physiol.* **12**, 200–209.

Zackheim, H. S., Krobock, E. and Langs, L. (1964). Cutaneous neoplasms in the rat produced by Grenz ray and 80 KV X-ray. *J. invest. Derm.* **43**, 519–534.

Zelickson, A. S. (1961). Normal human keratinization processes as demonstrated by electron microscopy. *J. invest. Derm.* **37**, 369–379.

Zelickson, A. S. and Hartmann, J. F. (1961). An electron microscopic study of human epidermis. *J. invest. Derm.* **36**, 65–72.

Zollner, G., Thauer, R. and Kaufmann, W. (1955). Der insensible Gewichtswerlust als Funktion der Unweltbedingungen. *Pflüg. Arch. ges. Physiol.* **208**, 261–273.

Index